DANCE
of
ONENESS

PRAISE FOR *DANCE OF ONENESS*

"*Dance of Oneness* is a masterful expression of how movement, ritual, poetry, and Divine Feminine wisdom can guide the soul into alignment with the deeper currents of life."

DEEPAK CHOPRA
bestselling author of *The Seven Spiritual Laws of Success*

"*Dance of Oneness* elevates dance to a mystical path of finding joy and wonder in every expression of life, but especially in the sacred design of our physical body. This book is pure inspiration. I loved every page."

CAROLYN MYSS
bestselling author of *Anatomy of the Spirit, Why People Don't Heal and How They Can, Sacred Contracts,* and *Invisible Acts of Power*

"*Dance of Oneness* is the most profound and sublime modality of sacred dance and embodiment on the planet and Banafsheh Sayyad is the greatest teacher of radiant embodiment I know. She has transformed my life and work and she will transform yours—with grace, mystical depth and tender, precise encouragement. This book is not only for everyone who wants to dance physically. It is also for everyone who now needs to dance inwardly to discover the marriage within all of us that births a new power and a new kind of human being."

ANDREW HARVEY
author of *The Hope* and *Son of Man*

"I will never forget the first time I saw Banafsheh dance. Not only was she wordlessly embodying every mystical tradition I had studied and practiced, but her dance invited me to fully inhabit my own body, marrying the sacred with the sensual, perennial wisdom with lived experience. In this brilliant book, Banafsheh shares her own compelling story of growing up in Iranian culture, with both its political tensions and its timeless beauty, and finding a spiral path toward the holy ground of dance. Then, step by joyous step, she leads us out onto the stage of our own life, where she sets us spinning in ecstasy and then settles us into sublime stillness."

MIRABAI STARR
author of *Wild Mercy* and *Ordinary Mysticism*

"If across the centuries Rumi and Martha Graham dreamt together to create a manifestation of sacred movement and divine wisdom in form, that being would be Banafsheh. *Dance of Oneness* lights the way into the depths of our own heart.

Here, no matter your age, skill, or background, you will find healing through Banafsheh's profound stories and simple embodied movement practices that brilliantly unites matter and spirit, healing and expression. I've been reading each page with tears in my eyes for the beauty and passion of Banafsheh bringing dance and the divine to all. This book will light a sacred fire in your belly and show you how to shine with reverence, playful power, and luminous joy."

HEATHERASH AMARA
bestselling author of *Warrior Goddess Training* and *Wild, Willing, and Wise*

"*Dance of Oneness* is an invaluable gift—part personal story, part spiritual map, part call to awaken. With courage, empathy, and poetic subtlety, Banafsheh Sayyad invites us to reclaim our bodies as temples, to dance ourselves whole, and to embody love as a living force in the world. This is not just a book about dance; it is a guide to becoming fully alive."

OMID ARABIAN
author of *The Universe in You*

"This truly marvelous book that could one day guide the creation of a new civilization, is a Teaching, an Illumination, a Revelation, that leads us to the discovery of who we are, why we are here and what we can consciously love and serve."

FROM THE FOREWORD BY ANNE BARING
author of *The Myth of the Goddess*

"How extraordinary that Banafsheh has been able to translate her embodied wisdom and divine physical movement into a book of words that compels us to dance. Dance of Oneness is both a 'how to manual' and mystical enchantment swirling us, lifting us, moving us towards each other and a new holy freedom. Read it and Dance Dance Dance."

V (FORMERLY EVE ENSLER)
bestselling author of *The Vagina Monologues* and *The Apology*

"In this profound and priceless book, the author describes an evolutionary pathway to the Divine Beloved. She reveals how she—only after high ups and very deep downs—succeeds in becoming a manifestation of the Divine, thereby integrating her experiences as dancer, yogic teacher and healer into ONE. This book is a milestone in the past and present of Sacred Dance, and can initiate its readers into the secrets of Divine Life inside a Conscious, Sacred and brilliantly Shining Body."

ANNINE VAN DER MEER
author of *Magdalene's Ascension*

"*Dance of Oneness* is an embodied cry for freedom! In a world that is becoming increasingly more artificial, Banafsheh Sayyad calls us back to the most authentic path there is: the path of the body. Not as a theoretical construct, but as a reverential experience that rebodies us of who we are. The practices that thread through this piece of art cannot help but bring you home to anything that got lost along the way—your feelings, your healings, your clarity as to why you are here. Practice doesn't always make perfect, but it does make presence. Engage with this book and its practices, and be here . . . again."

JEFF BROWN
author of *Hearticulations* and *In Trudeau's Kitchen*

"Banafsheh embodies beauty in motion. She has brought together many different traditions and modalities of dance into a single dance of oneness. Her dancing radiates the magnetism that oneness catalyzes in all of us who are dedicated to the pathway of love."

JIM GARRISON
founding CEO of Ubiquity University

"The task of our day is how to become divinely embodied human beings and Banafsheh is one of our most luminous guides for how to become the Beloved in motion!"

STEPHEN DINAN,
founding CEO of The Shift Network

"Dancing through the chakras with grace, power, and wisdom, Banafshch Sayyad has written a book that calls us to be the best version of ourselves—and that shows us the footsteps how. To dance in oneness rather than separation is to discover that the power of joy and connection dwarf the apparent potency of anger and hate. This is a book we need, right now—don't miss it!"

JEREMY DAVID ENGELS, PhD
professor of Communication and Ethics and author
of *On Mindful Democracy* and *Living Namaste*

DANCE
of
ONENESS

Embody Love and Luminosity
to Transform Your Life

Banafsheh Sayyad

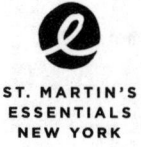

ST. MARTIN'S
ESSENTIALS
NEW YORK

Published by St. Martin's Essentials, an imprint of St. Martin's Publishing Group

www.stmartins.com

This book is not intended as a substitute for the medical recommendations of physicians, mental health professionals, or other health-care providers. Rather, it is intended to offer information to help the reader cooperate with physicians, mental health professionals, and health-care providers in a mutual quest for optimal well-being. We advise readers to carefully review and understand the ideas presented and to seek the advice of a qualified professional before attempting to use them.

Published 2026

Cover, jacket, and book design by Charli Barnes

Cover photo © Mehri Sahihi Modiri

Illustrations © Kate Tymoshchuk

Printed in the United States of America

BK07180

Library of Congress Cataloging-in-Publication Data

Names: Sayyad, Banafsheh, 1968- author
Title: Dance of oneness : embody love and luminosity to transform your life / Banafsheh Sayyad.
Description: Boulder, CO : Sounds True, 2026. | Includes bibliographical references.
Identifiers: LCCN 2025024738 (print) | LCCN 2025024739 (ebook) | ISBN 9781649633835
    trade paperback | ISBN 9781649633842 ebook
Subjects: LCSH: Dance—Psychological aspects | Dance—Religious aspects | Mind and body
Classification: LCC GV1588.5 .S299 2026 (print) | LCC GV1588.5 (ebook)
LC record available at https://lccn.loc.gov/2025024738
LC ebook record available at https://lccn.loc.gov/2025024739

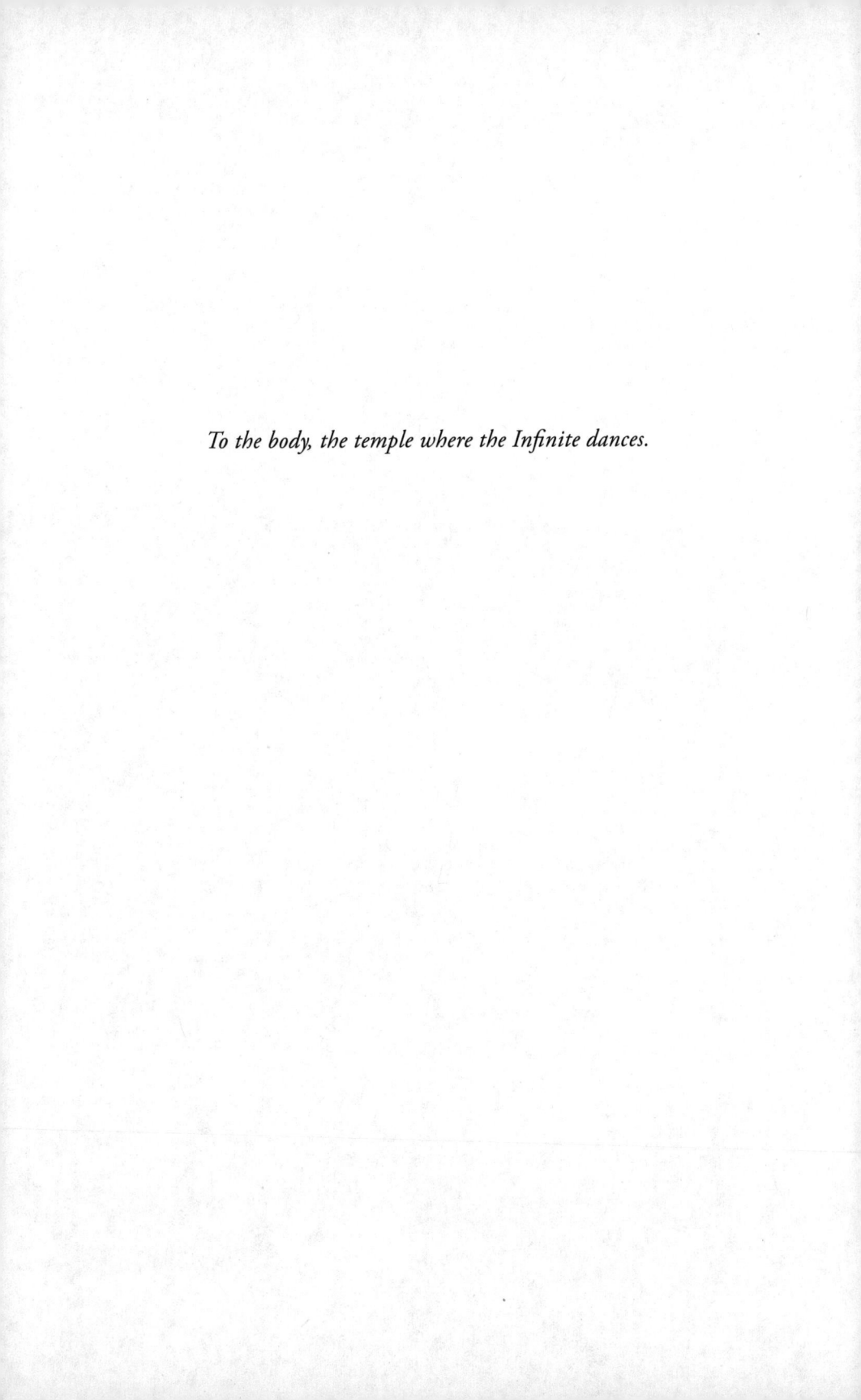

To the body, the temple where the Infinite dances.

CONTENTS

PRACTICES

Chapter 18

Chapter 19

 Scan the QR code to access the guided audio and video components that accompany the practices, or visit us.macmillan.com/danceofoneness.

FOREWORD

Andrew Harvey

Dance of Oneness is a one-of-a-kind and instant classic. Banafsheh Sayyad is not only the greatest living sacred dancer—she is to dance what Callas is to opera—but also our most skilled, exquisite, luminous guide into what she once described to me (as we were dancing in her LA apartment) as "Radiant Embodiment." There is no one like her and nothing like *Dance of Oneness*. I am so honoured to be able to celebrate here my amazing friend of 20 years and her continually astonishing achievement.

The only way I can imagine responding to the crystalline magnificence and tenderly ordered revelation of *Dance of Oneness* is to dance with what has been made clear and naked in my own soul. For many years I have been a devotee of Shiva the Golden Dancer, but it is only through my repeated readings of this book and my many astounding memories of Banafsheh's teaching that I find myself able to share what I am beginning to know at 73 about the Divine Dance that is simultaneously the nature of the universe and its greatest gift and challenge to us.

The One is both Nothing and Everything and the endless, intricate, constantly evolving Dance between the Two.

The transformations in the Nothing-Everything can never end. The Nothing is infinitely empty and pregnant at the same time and dances the Everything into perpetually astounding new configurations.

The One that is Nothing dances with the One that is Everything and all kinds of radiant evolutions streak from the dance like shooting stars.

All this would be amazing enough, but there is one more even more amazing truth and that is that each of us in all our ragged and crazy disguises are also One and have always been with the One. The aim of human life is to recognise this so you too can become the Golden Dancer. The Golden Dancer, the Warrior-Lover Midwife of a new humanity, a new creation and a new world.

Kabir, as always says it most concisely:

> *In the beginning,*
> *No "here" nor "there,"*
> *No "matter" nor "spirit."*
> *Only Love existed.*
> *What was then is now.*
> *This whole universe*
> *Is Love's endless dance.*
> *Since He showed me this,*
> *My heart keeps*
> *Blossoming in bliss.*

Don't fool yourself, however. You can know these all-transforming truths, but, as Banafsheh expresses in many trenchant and provocative ways throughout this book, these truths cannot become real and visceral until they are installed in every bone, muscle, and cell of your holy body and every gesture and caress of your increasingly divinized sexuality. The *Dance of Oneness* that Banafsheh has forged on her own unique path to radiant embodiment offers all of us what I believe is the single most powerful modality for realizing what Jesus in the Acts of John meant when he said as he danced with the disciples after the last supper, "The universe belongs to the dancer. If you don't dance, you don't know anything."

It has never been more important to receive the message, vision, and embodied truth Banafsheh's teachings and this glorious book open to us. Humanity is in the greatest, most terrifying, most potentially transformative evolutionary dance—the dance of Kali's global dark night. Her death and rebirth dance, her dance that is simultaneously a crucifixion and a resurrection. It is clear to many of us that this dance can only end in two ways—annihilation or the birth of an embodied, divine humanity. This vision has been known by all the great evolutionary mystics of all the traditions. Banafsheh and I, and many others all over the world, know that it is not an exaggeration or a fantasy but a reality that we are living.

In other words, the birth is happening right now in the middle of the obviously exploding, suicidal, and matricidal annihilation process. Extreme opposites are dancing Kali's Resurrection Dance together. Banafsheh's *Dance of Oneness* is Kali's exquisite gift to us of a carnal, divine, precise music in movement that can birth us into becoming dancers dancing in a new creation.

Do not even try to read this book once. I am on my third reading and am still awed by what is being revealed to me. Shockingly honest, brilliantly clear, nakedly and ravishingly written, peppered with simple but astonishingly powerful and penetrating practices, *Dance of Oneness* and Banafsheh's increasingly complete and initiatory teachings cannot be ignored by any serious seeker on any path.

Hosannas to Sounds True for its courage and wisdom to release this book in such a gorgeous and accessible form. Hosannas to Banafsheh Sayyad, Priestess and Rebel, Ancient and New, Empress and Slave, Sister and sublime Teacher for all she has suffered, imagined, dared, alchemized to offer us with such holy relentlessness, this and her living gold.

FOREWORD

Anne Baring, PhD (hons)

author of *The Dream of the Cosmos: A Quest
for the Soul* and *Divine Wisdom and The Holy
Spirit: The Forgotten Feminine Face of God*

Winchester, United Kingdom

"I just knew I had to dance. . . ." *Dance of Oneness* is an extraordinary book, written by an extraordinary woman, whose passionate longing to dance drew her to her life path and to discoveries that could enlighten all of us. These restore the sacredness of the body, and offer us the revelation of how the union of body, soul, and spirit through specific ancient rituals can lead to an ecstatic experience of union with the Divine Life that animates each one of us.

No book describes more comprehensively the tragic effects of the alienation from the body in Western civilization, reflected in the multiple illnesses, mental and physical, that afflict us. Understanding of the miraculous organism of the body grew as she followed this arduous path and discovered that her body was the key to the joyous union with spirit. She writes: "The body is the temple where the Infinite dances. . . . Only through becoming conscious in your body can you become whole and reclaim the deep, intuitive knowing that you are a spiritual being on a physical journey in this dance of life." Some spiritual traditions regard the body as an impediment to enlightenment, but Banafsheh reverses this belief, showing how the body is the key to that experience.

Interwoven with Rumi's exquisite strands of poetry, this beautifully written book is a Manual of the Alchemical Art of Transformation, with devotional practices and teachings that can illuminate and transform our lives. "Through joyful and painful years, hours, and moments, I discovered the Divine within myself, emerging from the spiralling fire of the dance." Hers is a book that heals the soul, so long banished by false religious beliefs from its joyous union with the body. Practices and meditations at intervals in the text are part of this process of healing which might be described as one of progressive illumination, leading to the reunion of body, soul, and spirit. Embodiment in the sense she describes it is a sacred marriage of matter and spirit, of the known with the unknown, the Above with the Below. "The key to this unity, the key to embodiment, is love."

Like Inanna of Sumerian myth, she made the journey into the underworld of her being, healing the deep wounds inflicted by cultural beliefs about women's designated place and role, indoctrinated into them by the flawed religious teachings of patriarchal cultures over millennia. Her journey shows us how to undo the beliefs and influences which have formed and conditioned us through thousands of years of patriarchy and, latterly, scientific materialism. In the decadent culture of the West, sexuality has become debased into a casual function instead of being the sacred and ecstatic rite it once was and could become again.

Her journey led her to make remarkable discoveries over many years, through her experience of different teachings and different forms of dance, learning and practicing Spanish Flamenco, Daoist Tai Chi, Chinese acupuncture, Gurdjieff's Fourth Way practices, the profound teachings of the Sufi Sages and finally, ancient Persian Whirling or Sama. "I wanted to uncover the earliest remnants of my culture, but didn't find any historical accounts of dance. I began to create movements and sequences by meditating on hymns and from my own imagination. I looked to ancient reliefs and artifacts for inspiration." She discovered that "just as the Divine is my Beloved, I am the Divine's beloved as well, and unless I see myself as the beloved of the Beloved, this love affair is only one way."

Over her seven years in the Gurdjieff Work, she received profound initiations, which she has distilled into five core teachings—offered to us as foundational elements that form the inner architecture of *Dance of Oneness*. These core teachings take us from a state of being virtually asleep—the current state of humanity—to a state of awakening, an awakening many of us are realizing, that is essential if we are to survive as a species.

While still immersed in her Gurdjieff training, she began to practice whirling. Whirling became her prayer and her communion with the Divine, "who felt more and more like my Beloved." She went to see a Sama or performance of whirling by the Mevlevi Order of San Francisco, a Sufi order dedicated to the tradition of whirling and this confirmed that she should follow this path, even if it conflicted with some Gurdjieff teachings. This path led her to witness a film of a Whirling performance by the Qaderi Dervishes of Kurdistan and to witness a performance by them in Madrid. This experience revealed that "The Sufi path to embodiment is illuminated through Sama (Whirling), expressed in seven fundamental initiations that form the foundation of *Dance of Oneness*."

In a key section of her book, she takes us up the Ladder of Ascent of eight chakras, illustrated with clear diagrams and culminating in the eighth chakra, our Soul Star and guide. Taking each chakra in turn, and relating them to specific rays of illumination, she shows us how to heal, through dance and meditation practices, the memories, experiences, fears and sorrows which may be impeding their optimal functioning. The end-result of this journey is Joy.

Her descriptions are breathtaking in their revelation of how we can heal ourselves through dance and discover the ecstatic experience of who we are as we engage through dance with the miracle of our body. Describing the Divine Feminine as the Great Mother, she describes how relating to Her as our Mother and as the Beloved, can transform our relationship with the Divine Ground. She says that this alchemical work activates a gamma wave within us that in turn "activates unity consciousness, the awareness of the quantum field of energy that connects us to all of life, known to the ancients as the Great Mother, who was known to spin, spiral, and weave the shimmering robe of life in which we live and through which we are connected to all cosmic life. . . . Imagine living with the concept that creation is an act of lovemaking and that you can extend this truth through the way you live your life as a dance. . . . We learn to make love with the whole of reality through our movements."

This truly marvelous book, which could one day guide the creation of a new civilization, is a Teaching, an Illumination, a Revelation, that leads us to the discovery of who we are, why we are here, and what we can consciously love and serve. "In a world where the sacred is misunderstood or undervalued, my mission remains clear: to help people unite spirit and matter through sacred dance, transforming not just movement, but life itself."

INTRODUCTION

An Invitation to Dance Your Life

Beloved dancer,

Dance of Oneness is an invitation to live your life as a dance—moving with joy, freedom, and an expansive perspective that unites body and soul and connects you with the greater web of life. As a Divine Feminine lineage, it awakens embodied presence and the wisdom of your soul, calling you to become a living expression of love. It is accessible to everyone, in every kind of body. You don't have to identify as a dancer to benefit from this journey. The guidance in these pages applies as much to how you live as to how you move. As long as you have a body, this invitation is for you.

And now, more than ever, this invitation is urgent. We are living in a time of great change and unraveling—old systems are collapsing, the Earth is crying out, and the soul of humanity is calling for a new way of being. This time of upheaval is also a time of possibility. It calls on each of us to awaken, to step into who we truly are—as channels for greater wisdom, the wisdom that can reveal new pathways out of our catastrophic predicament—and to embody love, not just for our own healing, but for the birthing of a new humanity.

It is important that we ground, center, and heed these urgent calls of our time from a peacefully responsible place where we can care for the greater well-being of one another because the personal and public spheres are one and the same—mirroring one another. As we live, and

1

with the way we live, we are creating the world. Instead of reacting and feeling like we are victims of the world, we can transition into being creators and co-creators. Dance makes us feel good, which leads us to want to joyfully connect with the world around us. It can free us from the shackles of the mind and the tyranny that exists in our world and help us remember that we are creative and love to create. The question is: What do you long to create?

Dance is one of the most profound ways to protest and manifest, as we saw in Iran from the earliest days of the Woman, Life, Freedom movement in 2022. Many people expressed what they were fighting *for* instead of against by dancing—for the freedom to dance is synonymous with the freedom to be. As we dance for what we love, we begin to feel the energy of what we love moving our bodies.

This opens us to joy. Instead of expressing anger at something, be it a friend, a relative, a situation, a so-called enemy, or an oppressive regime—and being consumed by that emotion—we channel our energy into what we love, into art, into dance. This expands what we love and dissolves what we "hate." While the movement did not bring about the immediate fall of the regime, it inspired important shifts and stirred the conscience of many Iranians around the world who had lost hope of ever freeing our beloved homeland, and it allowed us to hope again, which is a vital beginning to every story of triumph. This is the power of dance.

Dance is exhilarating, joyous, sacred, sexual, transformative, communal, and disruptive. It makes you whole. It gives you the necessary tools to align your body, heart, and mind with your very purpose for being alive, and it opens a spaciousness within you to see and live life from a larger perspective. Dance carries you inward to uncover your authentic self, and outward into rhythm and harmony with others.

From my earliest memory, I have been a dancer. My entire life has been a journey to uncover my authentic dance and create a path for myself and others that reveals the meaning of living an embodied life. My path emerged from both profound revelation and deep suffering. To learn the language of dance, I have been crushed and remade through a dance of opposites—extreme, terrible, holy, beautiful, and transfiguring.

This book emerges not only from personal devotion, but also from a deep response to this collective turning point in human history. It is a guide to becoming the kind of human being this era demands: grounded, awake, luminous, and guided by love. We are not here by accident. Each of us has a role in the transformation underway. *Dance of Oneness* is my offering toward this transformation.

I was born a dancer in a place—Tehran, Iran—where dancing was discouraged. Despite coming from a lineage of renowned male performing artists, my parents never considered dance training for me. In Iranian culture—as magnificent as it is—dance is not typically seen as a serious artistic path. This perception, influenced by Islamic views and intensified by the Islamic Revolution of 1979, has led to the banning of women's public dancing.

Yet I was determined to dance. For as long as I can remember, I have had two passions that remain precious to me today: one for the Divine, and the other for dance. These two flames merged over time, and dance became my way of communing with the mystery and a channel for the mystery to express itself in the world. This is the essence of *Dance of Oneness*.

This book shares the practical wisdom I've gained over decades of exploring movement and spirituality. It will help you inhabit your body with ease and joy, regardless of physical challenges, and activate light in your body so you can become a living channel of light and love. Even if you don't believe in the energetic or spiritual realm, wouldn't you like to feel more free, alive, and conscious in your body? Becoming conscious in your body will, literally, transform your life into a dance. As one of my greatest teachers, Jalal al-Din Rumi, whose verses and philosophy enrich this book, says, "Being in the body and conscious is cause for rapture!"[1]

Dance of Oneness does not require perfection. It calls for presence. The healing that comes through dance is often most profound when we let go of any ideas about how we should move or what we should look like. When we allow ourselves to simply be—to move in whatever way feels natural, authentic, and true—we find that we are already participating in the dance of life. The more we let go, the more we are healed.

If shame, pain, depression, or fear have kept you from the dance, let this be your invitation. These are extreme times. You are in need—and worthy—of the lasting joy that dance brings. Come into the dance and explore it with me, even if you have never allowed yourself to before. Dance with all your passion, with all of your pain, with all of your longing for love.

We do not need more perfection. We need more presence. More aliveness. More of us showing up in our bodies, whole and real. When we dance, we take a stand for life. We become a force of coherence. We reclaim our place in the sacred web of being. This is how we heal the world: not by fighting harder, but by loving deeper.

HOW THIS BOOK IS ORGANIZED

In writing this book, I have followed the sequence I use in teaching Dance of Oneness, guiding students to integrate the many facets of themselves into a unified whole.

The methodology of Dance of Oneness integrates three essential currents:

Wisdom teachings

Physical practices, including dance, to embody these teachings

Healing, which arises naturally from embodying wisdom teachings and allowing our knowing become our being

I've organized the book into three parts to make it easier to read and use.

Part I: The Story of Embodiment: Ocean in a Drop

In this part, I share my background and initiations into the spiritual, artistic, and metaphysical traditions that gave birth to Dance of Oneness as a Divine Feminine lineage. We will also explore what embodiment means and examine it through the lens of the Taoist and Sufi paths as living expressions of the Divine Feminine.

Part II: The Upward Spiral: Becoming Fully Human

The spiral is a central symbol in Dance of Oneness, representing the dynamic flow of energy both upward and downward through the body. Rooted in this sacred geometry, Dance of Oneness unfolds through thirteen luminous rays, or core principles of embodiment that initiate us into living love. In this section of the book, we will explore eleven of these rays.

To activate these rays, I offer simple yet powerful practices designed to help you clear physical, emotional, and mental blockages as you move upward through the chakras, or energy centers. These practices will support you in softening the armor held in different parts of the body. Divided into four sections aligned with the chakras, this part of the journey invites you into the magic of embodiment through dance and into the profound healing, expansion, and inner peace it can bring. We will also explore the dance and spiritual modalities that embody and integrate these rays.

Part III: The Downward Spiral: Becoming a Luminous Channel of Love

Having opened yourself in the upward spiral, you will activate the two final rays in the downward spiral. One ignites light in the body; the other, whirling—introduced in a few simple steps—offers the ultimate experience of embodiment: becoming living love.

THE ESSENTIAL REUNION OF BODY AND MIND

Most of us are disconnected from our bodies and unaware of the many issues that arise from this disconnection. This separation echoes religious systems that, for millennia, have deliberately denigrated the body as a vessel of sin. Most mystical traditions seek to transcend the body, and our modern culture values the mind over the body, leading us to adapt our bodies and senses to the demands of our techno-gadgets. As a result, we tend to live in our heads, disconnected from the wisdom of our bodies.

Dance of Oneness invites you to reclaim your body as the vital sacred temple that it is: the only vessel through which we experience all of life. Without the body, there is no religious experience, no mystical insights. Without the body, there can be no feats of the mind. Without the body, you wouldn't be reading these words. Only through becoming conscious in your body can you become whole and reclaim the deep, intuitive knowing that you are a spiritual being on a physical journey in this dance of life.

REALITY IS A DANCE

Throughout time, the mystics have told us that reality is a dance. The ancients created rituals to honor this truth, dancing the cosmic mysteries around their campfires. Through dance, our ancestors connected with spirit directly and when they combined it with music and drama, human spirituality found its first expression. Living your life as a dance gives you the tools to liberate your body so you can experience the sacred inner flame you were born to discover, regardless of your age or perceived physical limitations.

Like all other matter in the universe, our physical bodies are 99.9999 percent space or energy and interconnected with everything else. Yet we often define ourselves and our material world based on the tiny 0.0001 percent that appears solid. Rather than defining ourselves as being separated and isolated, we need to realize that our basic elements are forged in the hearts of stars.

Jalal al-Din Rumi inspires us to look at the truth that each of us is truly endless and infinite:

> You are not only a drop in the ocean.
> You are the entire ocean in a drop.[2]

I believe dance to be the only practice powerful enough to allow us to truly experience the interconnectedness of the universe in our flesh and bones. It gives us a direct visceral experience of the miracle of being alive, and it connects us with other beings in a meaningful way beyond words. If we can accept the invitation to dance our lives toward embodied love, dance can become the hope for our humanity.

True embodiment initiates you into experiencing yourself as a luminous channel of love for healing the Earth, restoring our bond with all its inhabitants, and helping to birth a new humanity that recognizes itself as part of a greater whole.

Dance of Oneness is a training to first become a well-balanced, responsive, and fully sane human being capable of dealing with all the conditions that life may present and to then become an impeccable lover, a wild and noble divine human being who can help heal our distressed world. In the words of one of my students, Dance of Oneness "resurrects the dead," breathing life back into a body deemed hopeless due to the ravages of the mind and emotions.

I invite you to join me in becoming more conscious in your body, allowing your soul's wisdom to guide the life you are meant to live. Step into the adventure of transforming your life into a dance. Or, as Rumi put it:

> *I've lit the garden with candles and set the table with wine and sweets.*
> *I've invited the musicians.*
> *My only wish is for your soul to partake and let your dance unfold . . .*[3]

PRACTICE

DANCE VISUALIZATION
with audio component

This simple practice can help you begin to connect to the rhythm of music and your own inner rhythms.

Select and play a piece of music you like that is five minutes long or longer.

Sit comfortably or lie down, close your eyes, and take a few slow, deep breaths through your nose.

Visualize yourself dancing to the music in a way that delights you—see yourself dancing well: confident, skilled, and free.

Notice what the dancing awakens in you—physically and emotionally—as if you were actually dancing right now.

Now, rise and "let your dance unfold," with your eyes open or closed.

Stop when the music ends—or after a few pieces if you feel inspired to continue—and tune into how you feel.

Welcome to the Dance!

∞

Remember to give yourself permission to put on your favorite music and dance regularly—especially when something challenging arises—and see what unfolds. Dancing freely allows you to move energy, shift your state of mind, and release tension. It can be a powerful way to process emotions, find clarity, and reconnect with joy. Rather than holding onto stress, let movement be your guide in transforming difficulty into flow. When more of us rise into joy without cause, we become the very wave that can transform the world.

love,

B

PART I

THE STORY OF EMBODIMENT

Ocean in a Drop

1

INITIATION

My Path to Dance and the Divine

Yeki bood, yeki nabood . . .
Once upon a time there was one and there was no one.
Beneath the azure dome, there was none but the Divine.
—THE CLASSIC OPENING OF IRANIAN STORIES

I was born in Tehran, Iran, in the revolutionary year of 1968 to two amazing people: my father, Parviz Sayyad—a magnificent actor, writer, and film director who became a legend in his own time—and my mother, Parvin Mahdabi, a force of nature, a beautiful woman, a lioness and queen, truthful, sensitive, and wise. I have been blessed with one sibling, my younger sister Maryam, with whom I share a very deep, loving bond as a fellow seeker on the Path.

I was twenty years old when I began receiving formal dance instruction. When people asked me where I had learned to dance before that, my response was always the same: "From the Divine." Over time, I came to understand that a dancer is an alchemist, and to become a dancer is to transform the lead of your life into radiant gold. The price of this work is non-negotiable: you must face your wounds and traumas nakedly as the most fundamental initiation into becoming your true self. As you journey through this book, I invite you to not only explore your relationship to dance and movement, but contemplate your relationship with your innermost self. Dance of Oneness can help you unveil your wounds and traumas—and glean their gifts—through dance and movement.

MY TWO PASSIONS FOR DANCE AND THE DIVINE

We each have a body, and every human being moves through space. Movement is the foundation of dance, and nobody is born more entitled to dance than anyone else. It is your birthright! You were born a dancer; we all were. Dance belongs to everyone, and nothing can prevent a determined dancer from finding their way.

As a girl in love with the Divine, I first saw Islam as the answer to my deep spiritual yearnings. My parents did not resonate with Islam, but my beloved grandmother, Batool Abedian Salimi—peace be upon her—introduced me to its fundamentals. For her, Islam was a disciplined path for cultivating compassion and kindness—the very essence of being human. She embodied these teachings daily: peaceful, loving, patient, generous, and compassionate to all. At night, she told me stories about the saints, filling me with awe, admiration, and a longing to uncover the mystery behind their lives.

She taught me the Islamic prayer, namaz, to be performed at dawn, midday, afternoon, sunset, and night. These prayers, aligned with the Earth's orbit of the sun, attuned me to nature's rhythm. She also guided me through the ritual of fasting annually. These practices became a joyful devotion to an greater unseen force. The steadfastness of praying regardless of circumstances instilled in me discipline and focus. From her, I inherited a deep devotion to Islam—one that would later give way to profound disappointment.

She also instilled in me a strong sense of community through visits to mosques and ceremonial gatherings. These experiences gave me a sense of belonging to a greater vision that was absent in the modernity of my school life. In communal ceremony, I discovered a sacred space where collective intention and reverence transcended words.

In this sacred container, I learned essential qualities: courage, friendship, steadfastness, loyalty, kindness, generosity, mercy, and warmth—values said to be intrinsic to Islam. Yet in the name of these very teachings, I witnessed hatred, pillage, lies, treachery, and even murder on the streets of my country before, during, and after the Islamic Revolution of 1979.

IN THE SHADOW OF THE ISLAMIC REVOLUTION

My parents embraced modern, secular Iran—a progressive, intellectually vibrant society striving to be on par with the West.

My father, an international celebrity, brought me into his world of film and theater, where I idolized his genius and humanitarian vision. In pre-revolutionary Iran, I spent much of my childhood on his film sets and backstage in the theater, immersed in his creative, pioneering spirit. He was like a superhero in my life—passionately dedicated to art, peace, and justice. His rich, artistic world and the extraordinary artists who inhabited it fascinated and inspired me.

A creative maverick, he rejected dogma and risked everything for his values. I saw how his limitless mind refused the oppressive shackles of ideology, and how he never compromised his principles for fame, status, wealth, political power, or even his own safety. Inspired by him, I felt called to be a pioneering artist, a radical freethinker, a risk-taker, and a maverick devoted to freedom, peace, and justice for all. Yet, my heart remained enchanted by my grandmother's simple spirituality. Though my parents were loving and open-minded, I felt that they didn't share my deep spiritual longings, and I often felt misunderstood.

In Iran, dance and music were stigmatized under religious influence, seen as subversive acts of liberation. Still I trained myself relentlessly, applying the discipline I had learned through namaz and fasting.

In 1978, when I was ten, my family moved to London after my father discovered that Savak, the Iranian secret service, planned to persecute him for criticizing the Shah's regime. Though we found comfort among Iranian friends who had also traveled to London, our hearts were still in Iran—where the Revolution was unfolding before our eyes on TV. My parents hoped we would one day return, but soon came the news that the new regime had confiscated my father's theater, branded him a heretic for his work, and issued a warrant for his arrest. His priceless original films and manuscripts were destroyed in the name of Islam—the faith I cherished—leaving me shattered by betrayal.

By late 1979, my father, sister, and I relocated to Detroit, Michigan, to live with my uncle during the Iran hostage crisis, while my mother returned to Iran. Trying to blend in, I adopted the name "Bonnie," but my British accent gave me away. My classmates accused me of being a spy, demanded I write to Khomeini to free the hostages, and bullied me relentlessly.

In 1980, unable to find work in the United States without a work permit, my father sent my sister and me to join our mother in Iran. The streets were thick with graffiti, fear, and hostility. Revolutionary Guards branded anyone who opposed them as infidels. Properties were confiscated, and dissenters faced imprisonment or execution. Our family's status as part of the old regime made us targets.

Soon, women were required to wear the hijab. At first, it was a choice some shopkeepers enforced, but gradually, it became mandatory everywhere—buses, offices, schools—until noncompliance led to severe punishments, including imprisonment and even acid attacks. Witnessing this erosion of civil rights was terrifying, a slow and calculated betrayal of women's freedom.

ADAB: A TRADITION OF RESPECT

When I was a child, my grandmother taught me one of the most important tenets of the Islamic tradition: adab (respect). "Respect and courtesy toward others regardless of their sex, faith, race, age, class, and station in life is the Islamic way," she would said. "Always remember to honor, love, and care for your neighbor as much as yourself." Even at the age of thirteen, I wondered how adab fit into the post-revolutionary Iran, because I could not see it anywhere.

Adab is a vast concept. Directly translated from Persian, it means "respect" and "courtesy," but its deeper, mystical meaning points to a way of being rooted in the recognition that there is a divine order and that all of life is sacred. In the Sufi path, to practice adab is to embody this recognition—treating all life with infinite respect and reverence, fusing the sacred and the secular into a single presence of humility and devotion.

My grandmother's profound adab shaped my vision of the world and became a compass for how I longed to live.

But when I returned to Iran in the early 1980s, I saw the opposite. I witnessed brutality toward women, and contempt for people based on culture, race, religion, and sexual orientation—all carried out in the name of Islam. I was devastated! Where were my grandmother's teachings? What had happened to them amidst the mayhem that erupted everywhere in Tehran and the other cities of my country?

I began to recognize the corruption of the mullahs (Islamic clergy). On the one hand, they imposed restrictions on people on the basis of religious ethics, and on the other, they led extremely self-serving, violent, and brutal covert operations most people knew about but didn't dare to bring up. I witnessed a complete and profound internal contradiction in the system and became deeply disturbed by what I saw, which was nothing but a drive for patriarchal power and control. And yet in my heart, I couldn't forsake my grandmother's teachings, and this created a painful conflict within me.

I felt I had no one to turn to. My grandmother consoled me the best she could, but her son and his girlfriend had just been lashed nearly to death by the Revolutionary Guards for breaking the new Sharia law that forbade any interaction between unmarried men and women, in private or in public. No words can describe how I felt when I saw the deep wounds carved on my uncle's back. He was the most gentle, creative, and sweet soul I had ever known. He said, "The Guards recited Bismillah al-Rahman al-Rahim (In the name of the One most compassionate, most merciful) as they landed their vicious lashes on me."

In horror, I thought, *This is mercy? This is compassion? Has adab died and is no more?* Bismillah al-Rahman al-Rahim had been a chant very dear to my heart—a heart that was now shattered into a thousand pieces. My beloved uncle Bahram—peace be upon his soul—took his own life some years later.

CALLED BY RUMI

Still only thirteen, I was desperate. I was beginning to question Islam as a faith I had cherished. None of the adults in my life could offer any real help. Then, one day, I encountered a book by Rumi. We had read and memorized his poems in school prior to the Revolution, but I didn't know much about him or his work. I took the volume off the shelf at our house and opened it. These were the first lines I read:

> You are water, but a whirlpool,
> flow onto us and merge with us,
> for we are the ever-flowing flood.[1]

I still remember the way the words lit up on the page and an electric current ran through my body. I felt, for an instant, as if the doors of my mind were flung open and there were no boundaries between me and the universe. All was one and flooded with light. Even at that age, I could grasp that this was an invitation—a real calling.

I had experienced many epiphanies in my short, yet deep spiritual life up until that moment. Slowly drinking the first glass of water at sunset after a whole day of fasting on Ramadan comes to mind. I could feel every cell of my body go into holy ecstatic rapture and begin to glow from receiving the water as if liquid light was moving through me. But somehow that and all my other epiphanies simply paled before those words of Rumi—or perhaps they'd prepared me for the encounter. I was immediately shown how rigid and paralyzed I had become from all that I had seen around me and not understood.

I felt that in telling me "you are water" and "we are the ever-flowing flood," I was being shown that this mysterious "we" and "I" are somehow related. One main difference between us was that I was alone, trying to find my way and purpose on my own. This made me a whirlpool closed onto myself. As all bodies of water are meant to flow into the greater ocean, I was being invited to flow and merge with the ever-flowing flood, to live my purpose in unison with the greater body of water alluded to in the poem. This vision filled me with a sense of peace and coherence.

From that day, Rumi became the central guide and friend of my path and my life. For me, his is the voice of love, a soul compass. Rumi's philosophy models a loving aliveness that doesn't get trampled, doesn't fade, and doesn't diminish with circumstances. This living love keeps growing and blossoming no matter what happens in the world, even in the face of devastation. It is unlimited love in action and a kind of faith that doesn't say, "My way or the highway" or "You must believe what I believe." It's the kind of faith that opens to universal love. In that moment of my young life, I had been blessed to meet not only the greatest mystical poet of the world as my guide, but also a saint who discovered, in the deepest sense, his way of being through dance!

Rumi will be a source of inspiration throughout this book. I will share passages of his poetry and teachings translated from Persian—by myself and others—and initiate you into the sacred practice of whirling that he popularized.

LEAVING IRAN, FOREVER IN MY HEART

In late 1982, after two and a half years in Iran, an opportunity to leave arose. Iranians were fleeing by the thousands, and the regime briefly allowed families of students abroad to join them. My father quickly enrolled at the City University of New York, and my mother, sister, and I flew to Vienna, then New York City, arriving just in time for New Year's Day of 1983.

Of the three of us, I struggled the most with leaving. After so many upheavals, I had at last found stability and friends I cherished. I also dreaded parting with my grandmother, and I carried warnings from my Iranian friends: "Watch out for the great Satan!" they teased, half-joking, convinced I'd lose my soul in the US. My harsh memories of Detroit only deepened my apprehension.

We reunited with my father in New York just as his latest film, *The Mission*—a poignant portrayal of post-Revolution exile—premiered to great critical acclaim and went on to win numerous awards. Not long after, We moved to Los Angeles, the heart of the Iranian exile community.

My family eventually settled in California, but life in the US was far from easy. We were often treated as "aliens" or even terrorists. I shared my parents' grief and the community's collective pain. Every day brought uncertainty—were we staying or going back? We clung to the hope of returning to Iran.

I longed for a role model who could bridge my Iranian roots, my passion for dance, and my vision of becoming the sacred, sensual woman I yearned to be. Instead, I found US media's portrayal of women to be degrading. It echoed, in an inverted way, the silencing of women I had experienced in patriarchal Iran. Both cultures reduced the feminine to an object for exploitation—whether through repression or through commodification.

In Los Angeles, my father began staging the plays he had written in exile, along with *The Mission*, which made him a target of the Islamic Republic. We soon learned from the FBI, who monitored us for years, that we could never return to Iran as long as the Islamic Republic was in power.

STEPPING INTO THE DANCE

In those days, the only topics of conversation among Iranians were politics and how we could save our homeland. Yet there were countless conflicting views. Everyone Iranian around us had been through some form of tragedy. While I empathized with them, I longed for respite from endless political debates. I was profoundly homesick—for Iran, for my grandmother, my friends, the street we lived on, my school, and every little thing that made up my life there.

I was twenty-one when I announced my decision to become a dancer. It came as an enormous shock for my family, even though I had been dancing since childhood. They asked me why it couldn't remain a hobby. I told them, "It will be my hobby, my career . . . and my everything." My father asked, "How could you possibly make a career in dance?!"—this from a man who had himself built a remarkable career in the performing arts. Most of my relatives praised my talent, but no one supported my decision to pursue it except my beloved sister. They said I needed to have started training as a child—something which was never available to me. Some of my relatives called dance a shameful profession that would disgrace our family name. I was on my own, with no support system, and no role models. I just knew I had to dance.

Very few women in Iranian history had dared to forge a career in dance. The dance I saw in my mind and felt in my heart had never existed. I longed to create dances that were mythic, spiritual, and poetic—works that would bring to the life the great Iranian stories and mythologies through beautiful, grand choreographies. When I tried to explain this, people looked at me as if I were delusional.

NECESSARY SACRIFICES

I knew my decision would require sacrifice, and it did. I chose to give up the approval of my family. I chose not to walk the favored "respectable path" for most Iranian women: earning a professional degree in law or medicine, marrying an educated and wealthy man, starting a family, and living a comfortable and privileged life. Eventually I enrolled in UCLA's MFA program for Dance, not only to legitimize my choice in dance as a career, but also to affirm Persian dance in the performing arts world.

Without realizing it then, the forms of movement I became drawn to were exactly what I needed to heal my wounds. Over time, I began to piece together my fragmented being. I discovered that breaking through to the real dance required me to start from where I was broken. Dance arises from a deep longing to know yourself—and to bring your authentic self to the dance, including the traumatized and shattered parts. To dance is to be destroyed again and again, and to be reborn again and again. It calls for continually abandoning the past for the purity of the present, with a commitment to stay transparent, authentic, and real.

Against all odds, this quest for the sacred in spirituality and dance led me to discover a unified mystical state, both in and through the body. In my search for a movement practice that could fully express the many facets of being human, I went on a profound, disciplined, and passionate journey through diverse movement modalities and spiritual paths. This journey ultimately crystallized into what I later formalized as Dance of Oneness.

THE JOURNEY OF DANCE

The forms of dance and movement I studied formally, along with those that flowered in me organically, all belong to sacred lineages that initiate us into activating the light of love in the body. The first form that truly spoke to my heart was flamenco—a ferocious expression that helped me bear the agony of my condition and begin to find freedom from the paralysis and silencing my traumas had inflicted. In flamenco, I discovered the lioness of the Divine ablaze with wild dignity—passionate and sensual, yet strong, noble, unapologetic, and unashamed of her power and beauty. This form gave me the ground to establish my identity as a strong woman.

My coming-of-age in Iran had been horrifying. The restrictions on the body, on freedom of expression, and on relations between men and women were so severe they could, perversely, make a woman want to disappear beneath a burka. In these circumstances, the natural process of becoming a woman was a traumatizing experience. Men would try to grab at me in public, and I began to hate the idea of becoming a woman, believing it was safer to hide. Today, to dance and embody sexuality with dignity—without blocking or censoring it—has been a profound personal journey, as has learning to wield the power of sexuality with responsibility and awareness.

This adventure in dance took me from the fiery flamenco to its polar opposite: the peaceful Tai Chi. I turned inward and touched the undifferentiated oneness from which all movement arises. The proud, distinctive lioness of the Divine needed to quietly merge into oneness with all that is. I began to learn the lessons of Tai Chi and how all movement needs to emerge from a foundation of peace.

My fascination with Tai Chi and the Tao led me to study Chinese medicine and become an acupuncturist. I longed to understand the body's inner workings and how to establish balance and radiant health.

My journey also took me into the Sufi path. I also spent several years in the Gurdjieff Work—an esoteric system of "working on oneself" developed by the early twentieth-century spiritual teacher George Ivanovich Gurdjieff who sought the "harmonious development of humanity" by uniting Eastern mysticism with Western science. In the Gurdjieff Work,

I learned sacred movements designed to bring mind, body, and heart into alignment.

It was whirling, however, that became the central practice uniting all my training and experience together. It flowered in me without guidance from anyone. As a child, I spun—as many do—but I never stopped. Whirling—spinning in devotion—became my primary form of meditation and the way I commune with the Divine. When I whirl, the "I" that I know dissolves into the unknown and reemerges as its messenger in the known.

Throughout this journey, I have received transmissions from the Divine Feminine. She has come to me in visions, in whispers, in the language of the body itself—each encounter a living teaching that continues to illuminate my path. These transmissions have woven themselves through every form and practice I delved into, revealing dance as a portal to embodied love.

Dance of Oneness is shaped by many streams—flamenco, Tai Chi, Gurdjieff Movements, whirling, Sufi teachings, Chinese medicine, trance, and Persian dance—all of them illumined and united by the living teachings and transmissions of the Divine Feminine. Yet it wasn't until I began to face and process the sorrow and shadow within myself and in the world that I was able to map the process of embodiment.

This chapter began the way all traditional Iranian tales begin: *Yeki bood, yeki nabood . . . Once upon a time there was one and there was no one.* Beneath the azure dome, there was none but the Divine. In the half-century since my birth, I have been on a journey beneath the azure dome, seeking union with the Divine. Through joyful and painful years, hours, and moments, I discovered the Divine within myself, emerging from the spiraling fire of the dance.

2

RADICAL EMBODIMENT

Modern Science, Sufi, and Taoist Paths to the Divine Feminine

My years of experience have taught me lessons in radical embodiment: True embodiment requires that we face and alchemize our shadow. Our body is already performing this miraculous alchemy—if we just tune in. So much of what we are looking for as the meaning of life is happening all the time inside us, if we just listen, feel, and attune to this internal dance. When we surrender to the alchemy of the dance, we become a crucible in which the shadow can be continually invited into the dance, processed, and allowed to offer its treasures of humility and compassion. In this way, we can embody our highest selves.

Sorrow brought me to my knees, pleading for a way to express what was needed amidst the chaos, horror, and cruelty of how we treat ourselves, each other, and the Earth. I prayed for the grace to become a vessel of love in the world, to serve the greater good, and to help people liberate themselves and become whole through their bodies. You cannot become whole without facing the horror and heartbreak of reality, and you cannot truly embody yourself without an ongoing integration of the shadow on all levels.

Dance is not only about feeling blissed out and flying into transcendent light—though it certainly has that dimension. It is about doing the radical work of embodiment, where you experience yourself as the marriage of spirit and matter, the marriage of the unknown with the known—your divine self and your shadow, all at once, simply, transparently, presently, right here, right now.

Embodiment is the union of body and soul, matter and energy, particle and wave, the inner and outer terrain. As above, so below; as within, so without. In this chapter, we will explore the role of duality in our understanding of the world around us and move toward unifying the forces of opposition, which is intrinsic to our dance.

Each one of us is an individual expression of the greater consciousness acting as us and through us, carrying our personal, familial, cultural, and global story. Embodiment is about becoming aware of the greater consciousness manifesting as us in form. It is about understanding that we are each a soul, an energy undertaking a physical journey toward wholeness, toward becoming living love. As the medieval Kabbalist Moses de León observed in the thirteenth century, it is exactly in this body and "by descending to this world, that the soul is perfected in all dimensions."[1]

Embodiment is about living our spiritual wholeness, the oneness and interconnectedness of all that is, through our individual selves and the body, recognizing and affirming that we are part of a living connected universe. Embodiment is radical because our default state as humans is one of fragmentation. We are conditioned to live in our minds, disconnected from our bodies, each other, and the greater web of life. We forget our innate wholeness, moving through the world as if we are separate, when in truth, we are threads in the vast, interwoven fabric of existence.

It is urgently necessary that we rediscover our interconnectedness with all of existence and the sacredness of life, as the present and future of our world depend on it. For the most part, our awareness is submerged in the mundane, day-to-day living, where most of us either experience life as harsh and merciless or we harshly and mercilessly try to control all possible aspects of life. Thoroughly identified with fulfilling the demands of our physical existence—making a living and attending to our basic needs—most of us either have no time or space to reflect on the sacred, or we delegate an hour here or there in our schedule for prayer, meditation, or other forms of remembrance. Today we see the result of this severed connection with the sacredness of life in extreme climate change, environmental and health catastrophes, and the extinction of species.

The level of violence, aggression, and intolerance in our societies also reflects this disconnect—the refusal to honor and revere life in all forms.

THE ROOTS OF SEPARATION FROM THE DIVINE

Our inability to live in sacred harmony with life didn't arise overnight. The separation of spirit and matter began four to five thousand years ago with the emergence of belief in a transcendent Father God. For societies influenced by Abrahamic traditions, this God exists outside creation, mirroring the masculine role in procreation, detached from direct nurturing. This dualistic view made equating creator and creation blasphemous, a belief I once held but now reject as the true blasphemy.

Before this shift, human understanding centered on the Mother Goddess, where life was considered sacred and interconnected. As Anne Baring and Jules Cashford write in *The Myth of the Goddess*:

> The Mother Goddess inspires a perception of the Universe as an organic, sacred whole, where humanity, Earth, and all life are interconnected as her children. In Paleolithic and Neolithic eras, the Mother Goddess was both the creator and the creation itself, rooted in the biology of a woman's body—nurturing and interconnected. Earth was seen as holy, human bodies as sacred, and all of nature as divine manifestations.[2]

The rise of monotheism fragmented this unity, withdrawing sanctity from Earth and body. Instead of harmony, division took hold, with life defined by opposites: death vs. life, good vs. evil. Monotheism positioned God as "spirit" dominating "nature," reducing the goddess to chaos to be mastered. This polarization intensified through Abrahamic religions and was imposed globally via colonialism, oppressing Indigenous worldviews.

God became aligned with light, creativity, and goodness; the goddess with darkness, chaos, and evil. The masculine came to be associated with spirit and transcendence, while the feminine was linked to nature and the material world. Religious teachings entrenched the separation of spirit from matter, intellect from intuition, and life from death. This opposition fragmented humanity's understanding, making unity nearly impossible without dissolving both poles.

Today, the Mother Goddess is largely ignored, yet without her, there's no balance in our understanding of life. This absence drives conquest and exploitation. If the physical world is deemed inferior, why do we pursue it with such relentless greed? We are a world profoundly out of balance. Restoring balance requires a return to the body, for it is through embodiment that we begin to reconnect with the wisdom of the Earth and the feminine—the living presence of the Mother Goddess within and around us.

OUR RELATIONSHIP WITH OUR BODIES

Embodiment begins with simply sensing and becoming aware of your body. In our day-to-day life, we are generally absent from our bodies, placing our awareness outside of ourselves. The source of this somatic disconnect runs deep.

Many spiritual and religious traditions, specifically those connected to Abrahamic religions—namely Judaism, Christianity, and Islam, but also Buddhism and Hinduism—have traditionally regarded the physical body as a cage for the unlimited soul and a "thing" to transcend if one wants to live a spiritual life. This view can engender hatred toward the body and prohibit real inquiry into our physiology, except when there is obvious disharmony or disease.

This disconnect has also been reinforced by secular thought and modern ideologies. Philosopher René Descartes famously declared, "I think, therefore I am,"[3] cementing a dualistic perspective that positioned the mind as separate from—and superior to—the body. This mechanistic view of existence was further amplified during the Scientific Revolution and the Industrial Era, where the body was increasingly regarded as a machine to be controlled, optimized, or transcended. In contemporary culture, this split persists through the glorification of intellect, productivity, and digital abstraction over embodied experience. From our increasing detachment from the rhythms of nature to the rise of artificial intelligence, we are subtly yet profoundly conditioned to live in our heads, often at the expense of fully inhabiting our bodies.

Many of us have inherited these worldviews—whether from religious traditions, philosophical doctrines, or modern cultural conditioning—and therefore don't know much about our bodies. We don't know very basic things like where our organs are and how they function. Some of us know more about our cars or our mobile phones than our own bodies! This may sound like a joke, but it is a real tragedy. Because here we are, these miraculous beings, and we talk endlessly about "knowing" ourselves, but we don't even know how our vital organs really function. Take a look at the general bias toward thought and emotion versus the body. We're so interested in understanding our psychological issues, but most of us don't even know where our intestines begin or how expansive our lungs really are. This terrible split between body and soul, splitting nature from the Divine, is an inheritance from patriarchy and specifically Abrahamic traditions.

When we talk about knowing ourselves, we typically talk about it only in mental, spiritual, and emotional terms. We either omit the body altogether in this equation, or we demonize it. Many of us are in the habit of saying things like, "My back is killing me," when it would be more accurate to say, "I'm killing my back with the way I hold poor posture most of the time, lift things in the wrong way, fail to exercise," and so forth. And when the body breaks down, we'll ask a doctor to "fix it." This seems to be our prevalent attitude, which I find extremely unhealthy. I, myself, suffer from this as well. A deep, broad re-patterning is required, and none of us are immune. We have lived with this kind of ignorance and body-illiteracy for thousands of years.

RECONNECTING WITH OURSELVES AND THE UNIVERSE

Writing about the Divine Feminine, authors Anne Baring and Andrew Harvey remind us that the system of dual oppositions that dominates our thinking "is only an arbitrary division based on the evolutionary experience of the separation from nature."[4] This division has helped humans develop individuality, self-awareness, and reflective thought as well as the power to develop technology and control the environment.

But having reaped the benefits of this evolutionary phase and standing at the brink of massive irreversible catastrophes, we are feeling the dire need to recover our lost relationship with nature and soul. The way to this recovery is through finding the Great Mother—manifest as Mother Earth—in ourselves.

For millennia, many of us only worshipped the absolute Godhead as the transcendent Father, and this has led to a tragic devaluation of nature, body, relationship, and sexuality. Now we need to attune ourselves to the Divine Feminine and dive into the nitty-gritty of how we live in harmony with Gaia, our Mother Earth—as one of her exalted manifestations— and blend the wisdom of the transcendent mystical systems that believe in "God" with the ancient worship of the Goddess. The key is to come in touch with the whole of life, both the transcendent and the immanent as one—one continuous flow of energy, one consciousness.

LIVING ONENESS: THE INTERSECTION OF SCIENCE AND MYSTICISM

Breakthroughs in science are paving the way for us to reunite with what we have become separated from so we can experience the oneness of all that is beyond the ways we have divided existence into little fragments. As cosmologist and healer Jude Currivan writes, "Science is beginning to rediscover the ancient insights that viewed the manifest universe as an all-pervasive cosmic mind. In this world-view, consciousness is not only present at all scales of existence, it is existence itself."[5]

There is a consensus among many physicists, astrophysicists, and cosmologists that consciousness, not matter, is the primary ground of reality; that the material world exists *within* consciousness. In his book *The Self-Aware Universe*, Amit Goswami states that "consciousness is the ground of all being, and quantum physics makes this as clear as daylight."[6]

Quantum physics asserts that it is consciousness that creates our reality and that everything exists in one continuous, unified field of energy, referred to as the vacuum or the quantum field. The quantum field is described as an invisible field of energy, frequency, vibration, and information that connects and organizes everything material and exists beyond space and time. It is the realm of consciousness.

These scientists view the universe as a living organism, with its visible and invisible dimensions woven together into a unified whole. What we take to be solid reality is, in fact, almost entirely space. The entire material world we perceive—including our own bodies—is only 0.0000001 percent solid, yet we devote nearly all our attention to this fraction. Even this tiny portion is not truly solid but composed of vibrating energy. And it is these subtle vibrations that give rise to the persistent illusion of separateness.

In reality, we are part of this incredible creation in which everything is interdependent on everything else. We are not separate from the dynamics that produce supernovas, stars, galaxies, universes, space-time, and the Planck scale. We are part of the flow of information, and what we call our body and the complexity of the biology all around us, the fractal nature of the trees and plants, are all an emergence of this information flow, including what we think of as our consciousness. "Everything is connected through space, and it is space that actually creates matter."[7]

With the discovery of the quantum field underlying our space-time reality, we find the idea returning—after four thousand years of neglecting the Divine Feminine—of a cosmic womb out of which all that we call reality arises and to which it may return. Dance of Oneness carries this lineage forward, embodying the Divine Feminine's call to reunite body and soul as one living spirit.

In this light, we can see that, embodiment is two-fold. One aspect is about becoming aware of the greater consciousness manifesting as us in form, and the other is about living the oneness—the unified field of being—through our senses. Both are ways of healing the long-standing division between spirit and matter that has shaped our worldview in the past five thousand years of patriarchy.

The key to this unity, the key to embodiment, is love.

Even though most of the mystical traditions we have inherited over the last five thousand years have reinforced polarization, we have also inherited less than a handful of traditions that understand and value the body and, therefore, guide us to realize the two-fold aim of embodiment. Each and every one of us contains within ourselves the entire history of human civilization. Our body contains about four octillion atoms. That's four with twenty-seven zeroes after it. An average of 200 billion atoms of everyone who has ever lived and died is a part of you, so you can access any knowledge, any wisdom, by tuning in and listening to the silent knowledge that can emerge when you become still enough to hear.

TAOISM AS A DIVINE FEMININE PATH OF EMBODIMENT

Taoism, dating back to 500 BCE China, reveals profound insights into the interconnectedness of all things and reflects the Divine Feminine in its reverence for nature, the body, and the flowing rhythms of life. Ancient Taoist sages observed and contemplated the body within the matrix of nature and the wider cosmos, the Tao. They recognized Chi, the universe's boundless energy, flowing through everything, linking all existence. This vision echoes Divine Feminine's wisdom—life as an interconnected web, honored not through domination but through attunement and flow.

These sages explored the body's terrain and its meaning, not by transcending it, but by journeying inward. Through meditation, they discovered energy pathways, or meridians, and their connections to specific organs. Remarkably patient and disciplined, they mapped these pathways with precision still upheld today. Their dedication and reverence for the body remain awe-inspiring, a testament to their deep embodiment and focus.

Despite modern advances in biology and anatomy, our understanding of the body pales compared to these ancient insights. Viewing the body as limited has been a pervasive, destructive belief, yet we inherit the potential for the same reverence and curiosity as the Taoist sages. Their legacy lives on in Chinese medicine and embodiment practices like Tai Chi.

For the Chinese, the Tao, meaning "the way," has two aspects: transcendence, or wu wei, and immanence, or yu wei (Tai Chi). The great Taoist sage Lao Tzu said, "The Tao is a well: used but never used up. It is like the eternal void: filled with infinite possibilities,"[8] and it moves like water. In this way, Taoism revives the Divine Feminine path of embodiment, honoring receptivity, flow, and the sacredness of the body as inseparable from the cosmos.

THE SUFI PATH AS A DIVINE FEMININE PATH OF EMBODIMENT

Another mystical tradition that can guide us into embodiment—echoing the wisdom of the Divine Feminine—is the Sufi path. While many regard Sufism as the esoteric heart of Islam, I will show later that its essence whispers from a far older source—the ancient streams of wisdom devoted to the Divine Feminine. Sufism emphasizes the inward search for the Divine through devotional practices such as chanting, music, poetry, and dance. The Sufi path centers on experiential knowing, rooted in the understanding that the only way to connect with the source of life and glimpse the mystery of existence is through an inner journey of awakening to love—one that blossoms into living love in the world.

Even though many Sufis, like most mystics, have viewed the body as a cage for the "pure" soul, as a woman mystic in the twenty-first century who resonates with Sufi teachings, I am called to reinterpret the core philosophy of this tradition from a feminine perspective. In doing so, I am evolving the tradition by affirming that we are meant to unify body and soul as one, and helping us remember its Zoroastrian, Mehri, or Mithraic roots, which honored the sacred union of matter and spirit.

The Sufi invitation is to live your relationship with the Divine—the whole of existence and life itself infused with the presence of the Divine—as a love affair. Through falling in love with the Divine as your Beloved, you begin to purify yourself physically and psychologically and transform everything in yourself that is not love into love. In other words, you aim to become empty of you and filled with the Beloved. You enter into a vast, boundless love relationship with the most passionate and ardent of Beloveds, who, as the tradition tells us, promises, "Walk toward me, and I will run toward you."[9] Imagine a relationship where your Beloved is even more eager and devoted to you than you are to them. What an extraordinary invitation!

Rabia, one of the few known women Sufis who lived during the eighth century, was the first person to call the Divine her "Beloved." She wrote the doctrine of Divine Love, which translates as *Eshghe Haghighi*. "The source of my suffering and loneliness is deep in my heart," she wrote. "This is a disease no doctor can cure. Only union with the Friend can cure it."[10] Only the Beloved was enough for her to work through all the contradictions of her life and find the alchemical transformation of her soul.

This divine love affair is all-encompassing and inclusive of lovemaking. Love is an all-or-nothing proposition. The invitation is to *experience* love in every aspect of your being and to *express* love with every aspect of your being.

Imagine living with the notion that creation is an act of love-making and that you can extend this truth through the way you live your life as a dance. Imagine that filling up the volume of your body with awareness is really receiving the Beloved. We touch, caress, and embrace the space around us with tenderness and passion as we learn to make love with the whole of reality through our movements.

GNOSIS

In Persian, the Sufi path is often referred to as "marefat," which means experiential knowing, a direct embodied knowing with your soul. Marefat draws on the idea of wisdom as insight and intuition. The Greek word "gnosis," which means knowledge in the sense of insight, understanding, and intuition based on participation of not merely the intellect but of the whole being, is what comes closest to marefat.

The first two central pillars and practices of the Sufi path are Sama and zikr, and they cultivate marefat. Sama in Arabic and Persian means "to listen." Sufi teachings, like many other mystical teachings, point to two kinds of listening. One is listening to the mundane world, and the other is listening to the spirit world, the voice of inner guidance.

When I use the word "Sama" in this book, I am primarily referring to the practice of whirling. While Sama refers to any of the practices in the Sufi path that engender this second kind of listening, ranging from seated silent meditation to whirling and wild, trance-like movement, it's most commonly known as whirling.

The second central practice, zikr—an Arabic word meaning "to remember"—refers to the chanting of the Divine Names in remembrance. In remembering the Divine, we connect to our own essence that is none other than divinity.

The third pillar of the Sufi path is adab[11]—the adoration of beauty in conduct, living with the awareness of and reverence for the sacredness of all life, and letting the "beauty you love be what you do,"[12] as Rumi says.

TRANSPARENT PRESENCE

Some say the word "Sufi" comes from the word "saaf" (pure, clear, transparent). Sufis polish their hearts, clearing them of all that is not love. The idea is that our essence is love and all we need to do is clear the debris of forgetfulness. This polishing is the Tarighat (practice, method). Love is the way to polish the heart, and love is the aim of this polishing.

The three main practices in the Sufi path develop a transparent, embodied presence in the *now*. Two of the practices, Sama and zikr, are ecstatic practices. Ecstasy means to be present in the moment. The Persian language guides us into this understanding. The word "haal" in Persian means both "ecstasy" and "the present moment." In both zikr and Sama, there is a fundamental experience of stillness and silence—a deep awareness of the column of peace that is at the core of every human being.

The Sufi path offers a sacred science that maps the soul's journey: from mineral to animal, to barely human, to fully human, and ultimately to divine human in a luminous body of light. Sama maps the journey from barely human to divine human. This is the path of a Darvish. The word "Darvish" is made up of two words rooted in the ancient language of Avesta. "Darv" comes from "darava," meaning "driver," and "ish" comes from "ushtra," meaning "light," as in Ishtar (star). This word becomes "ich" in German, meaning "I." So "light" and "I" are one and the same. Darvish, then, is "the driver of light," "the driver of I," "the carrier of light," "the radiant one."

RETURN TO THE DIVINE FEMININE

Both the Taoist and Sufi paths cultivate feminine, receptive powers within us and awaken us to our immanent divinity—the experience of the Beloved in our very cells.

The Taoist practice of Tai Chi guides us to attune ourselves to nature, honoring the Earth as a living being with whom we live in a constant exchange of energy. It teaches us to revere the interconnectedness of all that is as the foundation of our being and bring dualities into unity. Lao Tzu says, "Being is the mother of all things . . . know the male but keep to the female."[13]

For both Taoists and Sufis, movement lies at the heart of their philosophy and essential to embodiment. Embodiment through dance has been as integral to the Sufi path, especially the one Rumi illuminated, as it was to the Divine Feminine–based cultures. It was in dance that these cultures both worshipped and expressed the grace, beauty, passion, peace, wildness, and power of the Goddess. Dance is one of the essential ways we awaken to the presence of the Divine Feminine because it honors the body and the Earth, celebrating and embracing life in all its glory.

In light of modern science, particularly the discovery of the quantum field, we now understand that the universe itself might have emerged from a cosmic womb—a vast creative source. This perspective invites us to rediscover the feminine as a generative force not only within the dance of life, but as the very fabric of existence itself. Just as the word "matter" originates from the Latin "mater," meaning "mother," it is the Divine Feminine who guides us into the heart of embodiment, regardless of gender. As we dance, we attune ourselves to the cosmic rhythm—mirroring the cycles of creation and destruction, the wild and nurturing forces of the Divine Feminine—and honor the eternal flow of the universe.

The rebirth of the Goddess calls us to witness her in all her forms, to deepen our understanding of her ever-evolving presence, and to embrace the transformative power she holds for us and our world. As we embody the Goddess, we invite her wisdom and energy into our lives, allowing her to guide us in both our individual and collective awakening and transformation.

3

REBIRTH OF THE DIVINE FEMININE

Awakening to the Many Faces of the Goddess

The Goddess has been referred to throughout time by many names and faces: Gaia, Great Mother, Isis, Inanna, Durga, Kali, Aphrodite, Sophia, Mary are just some of her names. Although the tradition of the Divine Feminine was, over the past five to ten thousand years, replaced by patriarchy, she has never been destroyed. There is a part of her in each of us, regardless of gender.

Anne Baring and Andrew Harvey write, "The Divine Feminine is now initiating a crucial new phase in our evolution, urging us to discover a new ethic of responsibility toward our planet home, bringing us a new vision of the sacredness and unity of life."[1] She urges us to see her all around us, to hear her and feel her, and most importantly to *be* her. She is our Mother and speaks to each one of us in a different way. That is why there are so many representations of her. She comes in all forms and sizes, colors and ages. She is both our nature and nature herself.

Like most of us, I was not taught about the Divine Feminine by my family or culture. Yet as far back as I can remember, she has guided my life. She has spoken to me primarily through nature and dance, and she has communicated to others through my dance as well. Her presence became much more of a reality for me over time.

It is with complete adoration and praise that I invoke the Divine Feminine in dance and invite you to call to the one divinity of the many names and faces—Isis, Inanna, Durga, Kali, Gaia, Sophia, Mary—and in so doing turn to the one who is unconditionally loving, tender, gentle, beautiful, compassionate, wise, resilient, nurturing, terrible, and indestructible. We dance to remember her, letting our delicate yet fierce movement whisper, now roar, as we find our being again and again in her and as her. Through the dance of invoking the many faces of the Divine Feminine, we come through her grace to embody more and more of her many different forms, qualities, and messages. And in so doing, we gradually become whole and find our way home in this often estranged world.

MAY I ENTER? RESPECTING THE GODDESS

One of the most poignant experiences I had with the Divine Feminine took place on the Big Island of Hawaii. Swimming in the turbulent Pacific Ocean, I was tossed around by the waves, nearly crashing into jagged rocks but never quite hitting them. I had no choice but to surrender to the chaotic flow—into the wild, fierce beauty of the Divine Feminine. She was both exquisite and terrifying, loving and sensual, yet potentially destructive.

Sitting on the black rocks afterward, I felt blessed to be part of her vast queendom. Surrounded by luscious trees and flowers, feeling the warm rain on my skin, seeing the ocean rage in front of me with volcanic Pele passion, there was only oneness—material spirit, spiritual matter—the Earth as a living, breathing, celestial being: Sophia. I instinctively called this energy "she." From that moment, I always asked for permission when entering or leaving any sacred area on the islands. A Hula dancer later shared that it's an ancient custom to ask the Goddess for permission with the chant, "E hō mai?" (May I enter?)

In 2011, I taught a workshop called *Dancing the Divine Feminine* for the first time at Esalen Institute in California. My preparation included researching the lineage of the Divine Feminine, replete with the horror and agony, which made me weep without ceasing. I danced and wept for hours to uncover her in the wisdom stored in my body, yet I arrived at Esalen completely unprepared.

What unfolded was entirely unexpected. In our first group conversation, I found out that almost no one could say who the Divine Feminine was. The great disconnect from the Mother stared out from each neglected and lonely child hidden inside the adults in the room. The Mother's loving, compassionate presence was palpable among us. We invoked her in our wild, devotional dancing. In response, she appeared as a salve for each wounded heart, and all felt how their words and movement could give a most poignant and true healing expression to their pain. The most beautiful poetry and sublime dance came streaming forth—even from those with very little background in dance—transforming their stifled, numb, and paralyzed state around death into cathartic art.

What struck me and left me in awe from this experience was how the Divine Feminine reintroduced herself to this group of her children who had lost the way to her as the Mother who receives us when we die. Remembering her in this way, we began to reconstruct our fragmented selves. She revealed herself as the complete Mother—the Mother of both life and death. We come from her womb and return to her womb. In the vision of unity she offers, death is no longer the opposite of life nor a terrifying end, but an integral part of the great continuum.

In the early days of the Goddess-based cultures, there was no separate image of a terrible Goddess of death and destruction. The Divine Feminine holds the fullness of both light and darkness, representing the full spectrum of creation and transformation. She is the nurturing force of life, radiating love and compassion while also holding the mysteries of the unknown, guiding us through cycles of death, rebirth, and the integration of our shadow. In her light, she illuminates truth, beauty, and growth, while in her dark aspect, she invites us to face our fears, embrace our inner depths, and transform. This duality makes her both a fierce protector and a gentle healer, reminding us of the balance within all things. In her manifestation as Sophia, she is birthing a new humanity out of a great death.

SUFI/SOPHIA

Who is Sophia? The Greek philosopher Plato connected the word "sophia" with wisdom and coined "philosophy," meaning "love of wisdom."

In early Gnostic Christian theology, Sophia symbolized wisdom, the human soul, and the feminine aspects of God. As the womb of creation, Sophia brings worlds into being. The Gnostic myth personifies the human soul as Sophia, the daughter of the Great Mother. Losing touch with her heavenly origin, Sophia creates Earth in her sorrow and becomes trapped in the darkness beneath the light. This myth mirrors the human experience of separation from the source.

In this story, the human soul, a spark of the cosmic soul, is imprisoned in the body, disconnected and distressed. Becoming aware of this predicament and entering into gnosis can reconnect the soul with its cosmic origin. Sophia embodies both the Great Mother and the soul's longing to reunite with the greater field. Wisdom guides the way inward.

The Sufi path as a gnostic path draws on Sophia as the "soul of the world." I see the word "Sufi" as being derived from Sophia, and the path extends back to the traditions revering the Divine Feminine, drawing from the Mithraic, Zoroastrian, Judaic, Christian, and Islamic traditions, while also significantly shaping Islamic spirituality, infusing it with the language of love, the practice of inward refinement, and the emphasis on direct experience of the Divine. Its pillars—Sama (listening), zikr (remembrance), and adab (adoration of beauty)—are rooted in receptive, feminine qualities.

The majestic Hagia Sophia (translated as Holy Wisdom) in Istanbul, the principal cathedral of the Eastern Orthodox Church for one thousand years (which was later converted into a mosque by the Muslim Ottoman empire), is one of the great sites in Turkey—a land alive with the Sufi tradition and some of the greatest Goddess-based cultures from ancient times, one of which has been uncovered in the excavations of Çatalhöyük[2] near Konya, where the poet Rumi lived.

In the transformation of Hagia Sophia from a cathedral built in 537 AD to a mosque in 1453, the mosaics depicting Mary, Jesus, Christian saints, and angels were either removed or plastered over. By 1935, when Hagia Sophia was secularized and opened as a museum, much of the Christian iconography was uncovered through extensive restoration. The art of both Islam and Christianity began to co-exist side by side.

What I found striking in one of my visits to this sacred site is the image of Mary as Sophia sitting on the throne of wisdom, holding the child Jesus. It had been uncovered on the highest point of the apse. Without any premeditation or plan, this image now sits above the names of Allah (the One) and Muhammad, declaring the absolute sovereignty of the Mother of God and the progenitor of all that exists. It is worth noting that in Islam, nothing is above nor precedes Allah, who is considered "lam yalid va lam yulad" (he begets not, nor was he begotten),[3] yet we see the Divine Feminine as sovereign and the source of all.

In the Gnostic Christian literature, Sophia is referred to as: "Mother of All," "She Who Is Before All Things," "The Invisible Within the All," "Incorruptible Wisdom or Gnosis," and "Mystical Eternal Silence." She is seen as "The Feminine Godhead," "The Primal Virgin Mother, Consort of the Father God," "Holy Spirit," and "The White Dove." As the intercessor between the Creator and the created, as well as the light and the dark, she is the third force that connects spirit and matter.

SAMA, AS SEEN THROUGH THE LENS OF THE MYTH OF SOPHIA

The ceremony of Sama (whirling), which we will explore in depth later, unfolds in four stages—known as Salaams (greetings)—that mirror the journey of Sophia.

In the myth of Sophia, her children—humanity—have forgotten their heavenly origin, lost touch with their essence, and become entangled in chaos. Yet an inner longing—the spark of Mother Sophia—beckons us to awaken and return to our true selves. This yearning mirrors the Sufi mystery of *light upon light*, the mutual longing between lover and Beloved, as expressed by Rumi: "What you seek is seeking you."[4]

The First Salaam begins with the recognition that there is something greater beyond the chaos. By lifting our right arm up toward the sky, we acknowledge this unknown reality and assert, "Yes, it exists." When doubt breeds resistance, we shift our focus to Sophia, the greater light. By concentrating on essence, as Rumi urges, we sense the divine flow returning.

In the Second Salaam, we extend our left arm outward, as a symbol of witnessing Sophia in her creation. As we perceive her in all things, we reflect her qualities: becoming more willful, mindful, conscious, and loving. Divine intelligence—boundless and generous—begins to direct us, dissolving the illusion of separateness.

The Third Salaam marks a deeper unity with the Divine. As we feel less separation, differences like culture, gender, or age fade. Focusing on the Divine in all beings mirrors our own inner transformation, as the spark of light within merges with the greater light.

Finally, in the Fourth Salaam we begin to embody Sophia's wisdom and love in the world. The white garment of the whirling Darvish, representing both a shroud or burial cloth and a liberated dove, symbolizes the Holy Spirit of Sophia returning home. This stage is about living in service to the Divine, embodying our unique calling, and contributing to the evolutionary goal of consciousness.

SHEKINAH (FROM THE JEWISH KABBALAH)

Shekinah, from the Jewish mystical tradition of Kabbalah, represents the feminine face of the Divine and the indwelling presence within the world and our bodies. Her name means "the indwelling of the Divine" in Hebrew, and she is known as the "voice," "compassion," and "active presence" of the Divine, bridging the unknowable source and its manifestation in this world.

As Divine Wisdom and the Holy Spirit, Shekinah is both our physical body and animating spirit, embodying the Great Mother's stellar blueprint. Honoring Shekinah reveals our essence as living expressions of divine spirit, transforming how we view divinity, nature, and ourselves.

Anne Baring notes that "the Shekinah gives woman what she has lacked throughout the last two thousand years in western civilization—a sacred image of the Divine Feminine that is reflected at the human level in herself."[5] The Shekinah invites a sacred marriage of transcendent and immanent forces—a union of feminine and masculine energies within the One. As Kabir writes, "My Father is the absolute Godhead, my Mother the embodied Godhead, and I am their divine child, dancing for them both."[6] This eternal embrace of creation reflects a continuous act of divine unity and love.

THE DIVINE FEMININE IN ISLAM

While the presence of the Divine Feminine has been suppressed in all three Abrahamic religions, her power remains potent. The Quran and the entire Islamic tradition begin with "Bismillah al-Rahman al-Rahim," most commonly translated as "In the name of God, all compassionate, all merciful." The true meaning of this verse is "In the name of the One who births all existence from the womb of compassion and mercy." This phrase, one that so clearly invokes the feminine aspect of the godhead, begins 113 of 114 surahs of the Quran. "Rahman" and "Rahim" come from the Arabic root "rahm," which means both "womb" and "mercy."

Close to one-third of all instances of Rahman in the Quran appear in Surah 19, "Maryam," which centers on Mother Mary and refers to Jesus as a mercy from God to her. It is noteworthy that Mary is the only human being to whom a Surah is devoted in the entire Quran.

MARY, THE LIVING WOMB OF COMPASSION

Mary embodies Rahman through her compassion and mercy. She surrenders to the Beloved and gives birth to love. She is alive in every cell of the universe, a human mother as well as the Divine Mother, a friend, and an infinite comforter and consoler of the soul.

I became absorbed in Mother Mary's presence as one of the faces of the Divine Feminine several years ago, which eventually led me to Chartres. Notre-Dame de Chartres (the Cathedral of Our Lady at Chartres) in central France is regarded by many Catholics as Mother Mary's home on Earth. The twelfth-century edifice is a living sacred book replete with hidden truths and a magnificent labyrinth that is a vortex into timelessness. Since I first traveled to Chartres in the summer of 2016 to teach, I began to have profound experiences with the Divine Feminine as manifested through Mother Mary.

In my first visits to the Cathedral, I wept the entire time. I first felt shattered, then tenderly mended, embraced, and held. I felt I was being initiated into the fundamental technology of transformation: fana (annihilation, as in "dying before you die," in the Sufi tradition) and baqa (rebirth—life in the Divine that follows fana). It was a constant shedding, a death to the old parts of me. Death to all that is not love is necessary for your entire being to be inhabited by love—a dismembering in order to remember.

Over the years, I received four initiatory transmissions from the Divine Feminine in Chartres that have profoundly shaped both my life and Dance of Oneness. The first came in the Cathedral, while in meditation, when I received a transmission from Our Lady: "See me." Seeing Mary everywhere and in everyone became my living mantra. For months, I carried the Cathedral within me, and my life was infused with magic. Filled with love for her, the dance workshops I taught during the year that proceeded were imbued by her and references to her.

When I returned a year later to teach, I received a second transmission from Mother Mary: "Don't talk about me, be me." I took this profound transmission as guidance into my life, my work, and my art that year. In late 2017, as the world darkened with political turmoil and global suffering, I remained energized by Mary's presence, channeling unabashed adab, love, and goodness into my workshops and performances. But the weight of escalating environmental disasters, the killing of innocent people, and personal disappointment and injury eventually pulled me into despair. I was shown both the exaltation and degradation, the epiphany and the pain, that the Divine Feminine had experienced. I had entered a dark night of the soul. In that darkness, Rumi's poetry illuminated my path:

> I tried them all but none brought me more joy than
>   you. . . .
> My wisdom told me: fly away from the passengers of this
>   world,
> Why do you sit waiting with broken legs for your passenger
>   to arrive? . . .

Farewell to you, distressed body; you and to my regretful
*   heart—*
for until I was free of you both, the other heart would
*   not arrive[7]*

Rumi's words helped me see how how deeply I had become identified with what others think of me, to the point that I had lost a sense of myself. I realized I had been waiting, immobilized, like someone with broken legs, waiting for affirmation from others, who themselves are only passengers in this changing world.

Stripped to my core, I found myself saying farewell to my distressed body, loosening the attachment I had always held, and the habit of defining my well-being by how good I felt physically. Is it possible for us to feel good regardless of physical pain? The more I loosened the attachment to my body and the need to feel better, the more the pain diminished.

I was scheduled to perform at an event, but was in utter despair. My injury and exhaustion made dancing unbearable. Searching for inspiration, my eyes fell on a painting of Mary in my studio. "I'll dance to *Ave Maria*," I decided, choosing from the many beautiful versions of the piece. On the day of the event, I experienced a synchronicity. Two musicians I had never met before had planned to perform the same version of the song at the event. We quickly agreed to collaborate as a trio, with very little time to prepare.

As I danced, all my limitations in that moment—exhaustion, pain, the small stage—vanished. I felt like I was flying in Mother Mary's embrace. When the performance ended, the audience rose in a standing ovation. Grace had poured into me, healing my body and soul. Mary had transformed my breakdown into a breakthrough and shown me how, when we surrender to the Beloved, like she herself had done, transformative love is born.

In 2018, I returned to Chartres for the third time to teach and became aware of the most sacred time of the year in the city: the Feast of the Assumption of Mary on August 15. In 1950, in response to a petition signed by eight million people, Pope Pius XII issued a papal bull declaring the Assumption of the Virgin official doctrine, stating that "Mary was taken up body and soul into the glory of heaven." Four years later, in 1954, a papal encyclical proclaimed her "Queen of Heaven," bestowing on her the title once held by the Sumerian Goddess Inanna and the Egyptian Goddess Isis.[8]

Carl Jung believed Pope Pius XII's declaration of the Assumption of Mary as dogma marked the most important development in Christian theology in the last two hundred years. It was the first time in Western history that the transfiguration of matter had been recognized and the Feminine was blessed and sanctified. In Chartres, on the Feast of the Assumption, the Black Madonna is honored, symbolizing the continuity of the pre-Christian Goddesses with the post-Christian tradition of Mother Mary. A statue of her is carried in procession through the streets.

Witnessing this glorious Feast gave birth to my vision for a course called Madonna Rising. In that luminous moment, I received a third transmission: "Tell everyone to be me." When I asked for clarification, I heard: "I exist. All of the images and representations people have constructed of me are real. I am all of those manifestations. Tell everyone that whichever representation and image of me appeals to them and draws them—*be* it, embody it, emulate it, and let it guide you. This is how I teach you. Learn everything there is to know and feel about the aspect of me that draws you, from any tradition—whether it is the Sumerian Goddess Inanna, the Hindu Goddesses Durga and Kali, the Greek Goddess Aphrodite, Mother Mary, and so on. But remember, first you need to become present in your body, for your body is my temple."

Later that year, I received a fourth transmission: "Your body is your soul. Now is the time to embody Sekhmet, the Egyptian lioness-goddess —to claim your royalty as humans and to courageously free yourselves from every form of bondage and slavery: the old paradigms, the religious systems, and the institutions that have wreaked havoc upon this world. Enter into a sacred, holistic relationship with your body, with one another, with the Earth and all its community, as well interdimensional intelligences so you may stand in right relation and contribute harmoniously to the cosmic family."

One evening, I was blessed with the chance to be in the Cathedral at dusk, after hours, all by myself, arranged by a dear friend who worked there. I cannot truly put into words how it felt to stand inside that majesty alone. A profound silence filled the halls. That same friend invited me to dance and whirl in the labyrinth by myself, an invitation that felt like a call to reawaken the sacred geometry embedded in the stone through movement. I sensed I was participating in a mystical alignment, activating the labyrinth's latent power and verticalizing its energy—uniting Earth and Sky in a way that, to my knowledge, had not been done in that space for centuries. I became a student of the Cathedral, especially its labyrinth, and spent countless hours contemplating the deep mysteries of this sacred site, which mythologist Joseph Campbell called the womb of the world.

The labyrinth is an intricate, meandering path leading to a center, often unicursal, that requires concentration to find. In the Chartres Cathedral, it lies near the main Western entrance and is as old as the Cathedral itself, dating back to the thirteenth century. While this sacred form is embedded in Christianity, its roots are far older. The attitude of the Chartres clergy toward it is reflected in how they cover the labyrinth with chairs most of the time, opening it to the public only once a week. Before the 2000s, even this access was denied—the labyrinth had fallen completely out of use.

The more I whirled in the labyrinth, the more I surrendered and received energetic downloads. I sensed myself as a vertical channel of light stretching infinitely above and infinitely below—a current I came to call the "Vertical Infinity Axis."

As I whirled, multiple frequencies of the Divine Feminine began to emerge in correspondence with the chakras. One luminous resonance was Mary Magdalene. Others reached further back in time—the Egyptian Goddess Isis, Sophia, and the primal Mesopotamian Tiamat. During one Sama, I felt the entire Cathedral itself was the Black Madonna; in another, I became the Black Madonna at the labyrinth's center.

THE BLACK MADONNA

The Black Madonna is found across Europe, Turkey, Africa, and Asia. She is known as Tara in China, Kali in India, and Our Lady of Guadalupe in Mexico. She is Mother Africa and, in Sufi lore, a Black virgin at the heart of existence. She can be seen as the Egyptian Goddess Isis with baby Horus, her essence carried into Christianity as Mary, but embodying disowned aspects of the Goddess—fierce, potent, and transformative. The Black Madonna calls us into the dark, into mystery and depth, where illusions shatter and the true self emerges.

As the cosmic Mother, she holds the universe in her lap, symbolizing the void from which all life and light are born. She is also the Earth Mother, fecund and potent, embodying transformation, death, and rebirth. Uniting the cosmic and physical realms, she invites us to face pain and suffering, holding and guiding us through it.

MARY MAGDALENE, THE INVISIBLE TOWER OF THE SUFI PATH

Mother Mary unites with the Beloved to birth the divine child, modeling divine love and surrender. Yet it is Mary Magdalene—Miryam in Aramaic—who shows us how to love the Beloved through loving another human being. Miryam and Yeshua (Jesus) shared a transformative love that nurtured mutual evolution. We now know that Miryam was the beloved companion and wife of Yeshua, the mother of his children, and co-teacher with him in Palestine.

Yeshua referred to her as the woman who "Knew The All." She has been called a full spectrum of names—from prostitute and repentant sinner to priestess in the Isis tradition, the most important single teacher in the early Christian movement aside from Yeshua, and the carrier of the Divine Feminine counterpart to the Divine Masculine embodied by him.

Miryam, often shrouded in mystery, communicates through dreams, meditation, and visions, helping us remember her, and in doing so, remember ourselves. As the living embodiment of Yeshua's teachings, she has been called "The Apostle of Apostles" and "The Tower of Wisdom." Her title, "Magdalene," comes from "Migdala," meaning "tower" in

Aramaic. Yeshua proclaimed, "When all have abandoned me, only she shall stand beside me like a tower. From this day forth, she shall be known as Migdalah, for she shall be as a tower to my flock, and the time will soon come when her tower shall stand alone by mine."[9]

Miryam calls us into wholeness through love, holding us through the valleys of loss, fear, and uncertainty. With a healing balm at her heart, she offers renewal through the alchemical waters of love. She invites us to open our hearts to trust, to love, and to awaken to the beauty within and all around us.

Miryam teaches strength woven with compassion, urging us to witness the beauty and goodness of the world with open hearts—even amidst chaos. She embodies the courage to speak truth with love and dignity, her voice like honey—nourishing and sweet. Unbound and liberated, Miryam carries the energy of Aphrodite, Goddess of Love, Beauty, and Eros, showing us how trust and surrender in love open a gateway to the infinite. Often depicted with flowing hair, she unites the sensual and the sacred. Her symbols—the anchor and the heart—inspire us to root in courage and live in service to beauty, truth, and goodness. Miryam reminds us that every choice has consequences, calling us to act in alignment with our heart's deepest knowing. She invites us to follow the tears of compassion and surrender to grace, allowing them to heal, transform, and lead us to the Beloved.

Although Miryam is not explicitly referenced in Sufi texts, her role as a revered teacher of the Gnostics suggests that she may also be understood as a spiritual foremother of the Sufi tradition, which is fundamentally a gnostic path. Her teachings—centered on intimate union with the Beloved and the embodiment of divine love—resonate deeply with Sufi principles, as does the ideal of the Anthropos, "the fully awakened human being." The Sufis call the Divine Doost the "Friend," and Miryam, often called "friend" by her followers, shares this spirit. In essence, Miryam embodies the qualities of a Darvish—a true friend of the Friend. She is also said to carry the radiant frequency of Sophia.

DIVINE FEMININE ROLE MODELS

The Divine Feminine path of embodiment is about uniting the sensual and the sacred, blending the great sensual powers of Aphrodite, the Goddess of Love, Beauty, and Eros with the great loving powers of Mother Mary. Yet the living experience of the Goddess isn't complete without a third presence: Sophia, *embodied wisdom*. She, as wisdom, links the dyad of Aphrodite and Mary to form the triad: eros, love, and wisdom.

To give form and manifestation to this triad, a fourth presence is needed: a woman who, by embodying—Aphrodite, Mary, and Sophia— gives birth to herself in the full glory of an embodied woman, living the timeless feminine triad in the world. Miryam, the Migdala, was such a woman and models this living embodiment for us. What I love about this quartet is that it opens a pathway for women to access the beauty, rapture, and wisdom of the timeless feminine.

People often ask me, "How can I learn to embody the Divine Feminine?" My answer is: You learn it from everything and every-where, and especially from the Earth herself. She is always present, even when people and circumstances seem to be explicitly suppressing her. When Rumi says, "I didn't see anyone who had complete devo-tion, so I learned devotion from devotion itself,"[10] he means he learned from the *idea* of devotion. In the same way, I learned about the Divine Feminine both from the idea of her and from her countless manifes-tations across cultures and time. She revealed herself to me primarily through nature and sacred sites, but also through art, music, cities, sto-ries, world events, people, and feminine icons like Marilyn Monroe, Marlene Dietrich, Joan of Arc, Rabia, the heroic Iranian saint Tahereh Qurrat al-Ayn, and countless others.

I saw the Divine Feminine in my grandmother—peace be upon her—who had been denied formal education because, in her time, girls were not considered "important enough" to teach. Their destinies, at best, were to become mothers and housewives. Yet, my grandmother grew up to be an incredibly wise woman in addition to being a mother and housewife. She sometimes wore the hijab and other times she did not. I once asked her, "Maman joon (dear mother), are you Mohajab (a veiled woman) or not?" And she said, "I wear the hijab when I feel like it. When I want to be in my own private space or don't feel like dressing up and doing my hair but still need to go out in public, I wear it. That way, I'm like a shadow moving among people, unrecognized. Other times, when I feel beautiful and my hair is done, I choose not to wear it."

I love that response because, in essence, she was saying, "Conditions don't rule me. I use them to birth my own identity." This freedom, however, belonged to a time before the hijab became mandatory in Iran, when women were stripped of the right to choose for themselves. My grandfather—peace be upon him—was very strong and authoritarian. As far as I know, my grandmother bore his aggression and frequent outbursts with an incredibly accommodating silence throughout her life with him. From her I learned patience, but I also sensed a kind of complacency and passivity. So I sought the Divine Feminine qualities of strength, valiance, and courage elsewhere.

My mother, who is a truly amazing, passionate, and witty woman, also models important aspects of the Divine Feminine for me. But I admit, it took me a while to see her in this light. Like many mother-daughter relationships, ours was fraught with struggle. By nature, I was quieter and more introverted, preferring to move at a slower, more contemplative rhythm, while she lived in a rapid, fiery tempo, fueled by her abundant energy.

I have to confess that I also had a bias against women. As a teen, I preferred the company of my father's circle of friends. His friends were brilliant artists, intellectuals, actors, writers, filmmakers, poets, and musicians. I enjoyed listening to their philosophical conversations which often revolved around film, literature, art, and music.

In contrast, my mother's circles often centered around recipes, fashion, and gossip—none of which interested me. Looking back, I realize this reflected my own patriarchal bias, the belief that women were "just not that smart." Over time I questioned whether this was truly my belief, or if I had been conditioned to think that way as an "Athena type"—the "good girl" enamored with her father. In Greek mythology, Athena was born from the head of Zeus, embodying the archetype of intellectually driven women who are more in touch with their masculine side than their feminine. Many women, especially those who are career-minded in the West, carry a strong Athena imprint.

With time, I grew to appreciate and love my mother's way of being. This shift came through sincere inquiry into why I had struggled with her so much. I realized that I mistrusted and judged the part of myself she reflected back to me—the part that is simply about being, radiating beauty, and living by intuition rather than being overtly analytical. To reconcile with her, I had to heal the masculine disdain for the feminine within myself. I invite you to contemplate how those around you reflect different aspects of the Divine Feminine, and to consider how you embody the Divine Feminine—often without even realizing it.

PRACTICE

VISUALIZING THE DIVINE FEMININE AS THE GREAT MOTHER
with audio component

I invite you to enter this practice of communion with the Divine Mother. Let us adore the Mother of all—her living presence here in this dimension, dwelling within us and among us in the midst of her queendom, available to all who seek her. Often unknown and unrecognized, she works quietly in the depths of life, opening us to the reality of her presence and to the sacredness of creation: love, justice, wisdom, and truth.

> Settle into a comfortable position. Close your eyes, and gently turn your awareness inward. Take three deep breaths in and out through your nose, allowing each breath to anchor you deeper into presence.

> Call upon the Divine Mother. Allow her to come to you in whatever way she chooses. She is known by many names and

countless images, appearing through the ages in forms each culture could most readily recognize. Feel her presence and open your heart to embrace her. She has a thousand and one names, a thousand and one skin tones, and shines in a thousand and one adornments.

Call her by the name that opens your heart, the name that flows most naturally to your lips. If no name comes, wait and listen—she will whisper one to you. Call to her in your mother tongue or the language of your soul: Mother, Mama, Maman, Madre, Maadar, Mutter, Um, Aane, Gaia, Mary, Isis, Inanna, Durga, Shekinah, Sophia or any of her countless sacred names, each a doorway to her presence.

Pour your love into her as you rest in her embrace. Know that you can turn to her at any moment, for you never fall outside her embrace. Let the trust born of this knowing resonate through your whole body as you say:

> "Holy Mother, I know you love me, and I love you.
>
> Show me how to live in harmony with you.
>
> Guide me to be your messenger."

Stay in this presence for as long as you wish. When you are ready to close the practice, take three deep breaths through your nose, and open your eyes from the deep presence and communion you have experienced with the Divine Mother.

Look around you and behold her beneficence, her glorious beauty, manifested everywhere, in everyone, and in yourself.

∞

With a foundation in the meaning of embodiment, you are now ready to bring these teachings into your body and begin the journey of becoming fully human.

PART II

THE UPWARD SPIRAL

Becoming Fully Human

SECTION 1

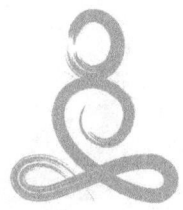

The Journey Begins

Mapping the Upward Spiral

4

THE SUN OF LOVE

Dance of Oneness Map
to Embodiment

We now begin our practical journey of embodiment, discovering what it means to be fully human. As you ascend the upward spiral, I invite you to shed the layers that hide your luminous essence and step more fully into who you truly are.

The most extraordinary thing in life is reality itself—with all its so-called "ordinariness" and ups and downs. To get real as individual expressions of the greater consciousness—as souls living on Earth—is profoundly challenging. It requires cultivating a pragmatic spirituality that helps us drop the masks and all that prevents us from showing up in integrity—which, in truth, is nearly everything that characterizes life today.

More than ever, the demand of our time is to get real and show up fully in service to love, in harmony with the Earth. We are at the brink of extinction. We, as a collective, have not been contributing harmoniously to life on our planet. Just as cancer takes hold when individual cells fall out of harmony with the body and act as if they were separate entities, most of us feel separate from the Earth and from one another, creating a condition akin to cancer that endangers the planet and all life. Dance and movement can help us re-align our body, heart, and mind with the Earth and with one another, opening us to bear the light of love in these intense times—putting love into action to help birth a new humanity.

THE SUN OF LOVE

Over the next few chapters, I will introduce you to the thirteen rays of Dance of Oneness that initiate you into living love through practices that serve both what I call "Art Dancers" (professional dancers and dance students) and "Life Dancers" (those who live their lives as a dance). Based on the premise that the "universe is a dance," these initiatory teachings—weaving the art of embodiment through dance, wisdom teachings, and healing—prepare you to live your life as a graceful dance during these dire times.

In Dance of Oneness, we move to create spaciousness inside so we can become luminous channels of love—great flames—emanating from the sun. Mehr, the divine presence ancient Iranians revered—also known as Mithra—means the sun, the divinity of light, as well as love and covenant. Mehr is the sun whose light shines not only upon the outer world but also within the heart. It is divine love, dissolving boundaries, asking nothing in return, flowing simply because it must—like the sun rising each day without questioning who is worthy of its warmth.

As Rumi says, "The sun shines because it is in love."[1] Its emanations are the expression of love. We, too, are continually showered by love—sometimes intense, sometimes tender—but always vital. Without it, we would perish. In the same way sunlight radiates from the sun as an expression of its love, we too can radiate light through our loving. Love is not the same as light, but it expands and magnifies it. Even darkness gravitates toward love, for at the core of all existence lies the longing to love and be loved.

As we move through the thirteen rays of Dance of Oneness, remember: each is essential—none greater or lesser than the others.

ACTIVATE THE LIGHT OF LOVE

As an individual expression of the greater consciousness, you are a being of light—love made manifest. This journey invites you to remember who you are, and why you are here. You will be guided to explore the places within you where light cannot yet reach—where old beliefs, pain, and fear have hardened into density and rigidity. These very places reveal your soul's work: to open, soften, and expand into more light, into more love.

The more light you are able to hold and radiate, the higher the frequency of your being and the greater your level of consciousness. As you heal and re-pattern ailments, limiting beliefs, and fragmentation, you access your light body more fully. In doing so, you begin to sustain a state of empowerment—a joyful, embodied love that infuses your heart, body, and mind. You become a light unto yourself, a living embodiment of love, opening your wings to fly.

Ray 1: Presence Begins in the Body

As inscribed on the facade of the Temple of Luxor in Egypt: "The body is the house of God"[2] and "Man, know thyself, and you are going to know the gods."[3]

As long as you are in a body, presence begins with becoming conscious in your body. Thoughts and emotions can easily pull you into the past or propel you into the future, but your body is always here, now. The gateway to presence in the now is through sensing and filling up the volume of your body with loving awareness—with consciousness, energy, soul, or Chi.

PRACTICE

BASIC MEDITATION
with audio component

This practice will help you become conscious in your body. I recommend doing it for ten to forty-five minutes every morning upon waking. If you are new to meditation, begin with ten minutes and gradually increase to forty-five.

Time required: 10-45 minutes

Create a sacred space—a quiet sanctuary where you can return each day for your meditation practice. Sit comfortably, whether cross-legged, kneeling on the ground, or on a chair. If you sit on a chair, place both feet flat on the ground and feel the Earth supporting you. If you sit cross-legged or kneeling, be sure your knees are lower than your pelvis. Place a zafu (meditation cushion) or any firm cushion beneath you so your tailbone rests comfortably and your posture is upright. Let your knees drop below your pelvis, your chest rest directly above your pelvis, and your neck align naturally above your chest.

Throughout the meditation, direct your awareness inward to each body part and concentrate gently on that area. I will guide you to progressively awaken presence in your body, beginning with your navel. Try not to form a visual image of the body part in your mind. Instead, bring your attention directly into the area I indicate. If you notice yourself imagining it, simply re-center and return your awareness to the felt sense of that body part. Take slow, deep breaths in and out through your nose, pausing gently before each new in-breath, until your body naturally asks for another.

Begin by placing the back of your left hand in your right hand, with the tips of your thumbs touching. Let your hands rest on your lap, and close your eyes. Take a deep breath in through your nose, and exhale through your nose. Pause in the stillness before your next breath.

Take another deep breath, expanding your chest and upper back as you inhale. Slowly exhale. As you pause before your next in-breath, bring your awareness to your navel.

As you inhale, let your belly rise—expanding your abdomen outward. As you exhale, allow your abdomen to soften inward, relaxing your buttocks and letting your pelvis and hips settle fully onto the surface beneath you. Pause gently before your next in-breath. With each breath, continue expanding as you inhale and softening as you exhale.

Take another deep breath and expand your abdomen in the area of your navel. Exhale slowly. Pause in the stillness before your body calls for the next breath, sensing your legs come alive from within. Feel energy moving down from your hips through your thighs, knees, shins, calves, and ankles into your feet. Sense your toes.

Take another deep breath and expand your whole torso as you inhale, rising from your navel area up into your abdomen and chest. As you exhale, relax your shoulders. In the gentle pause before your next in-breath, sense your arms coming alive from within. Feel your upper arms, elbows, forearms, wrists, and hands. Sense your fingers.

Take another deep breath, expanding your whole torso as you inhale. As you exhale, soften your neck. Rest for a moment in the stillness before your body naturally calls for the next breath, and trace your spine with awareness, from the base of your skull down to your tailbone, becoming present in your upper, middle, and lower back.

Take another deep breath, expanding your whole torso as you inhale. Exhale slowly. As you pause gently before your next in-breath, become aware of your face. Sense the top of your head, then soften your forehead, eye sockets, temples, cheeks, jaw, and chin. Relax your lips, feeling them soft and kissable.

Take another deep breath and sense your whole body expanding as you inhale. As you exhale, ease your weight into the chair or cushion, and feel the living Earth through the soles of your feet and your legs (if you are seated on the ground). Pause in the stillness and sense your whole body sitting here now. Touch into the global sensation of your body and feel a harmonious distribution of energy throughout. Allow your mind to grow quiet and still.

Continue taking slow, deep breaths. With each breath, feel your body growing more and more relaxed, your mind becoming more and more still. Stay in the silence and listen. Allow every sound inside and outside to simply be. Do not resist, do not defend. When thoughts enter your mind, do not fight them—simply observe and let them pass. Flow with your breath and feel yourself, simply and effortlessly, here now. As you inhale, create more volume and spaciousness within your body. As you exhale, release tightness, rigidity, and any constriction. Soften and open the places that resist spaciousness. In the gentle pause before your next in-breath, feel the stillness growing within you.

Now you are ready for an invocation:

In the name of the One, endlessly expanding mystery—all and everything, and no-thing—fill the temple of my heart, mind, and body with your radiant presence, that I may align with the radiance of my soul. Let me remember myself as a unique expression of you in form, and inspire others to awaken to this remembrance within themselves. Guide me to walk as your messenger of compassion, mercy, and loving discernment upon the Earth, in harmony with her rhythms and in service to her wholeness.

Flow with your breath, soften the edges and boundaries of your body. Feel yourself gradually dissolving into pure energy, beginning with your head, then moving progressively down your face, neck, shoulders, arms, and hands, your chest and abdomen, your hips, legs, feet, and toes.

Remember: your body is 99.9999 percent energy. Flow with your breath and sense yourself merging with the energy of the greater space around you. Stay in this presence for as long as you can—at least five to ten minutes. Feel yourself as pure consciousness, as awareness—as loving awareness.

When you are ready to bring your meditation to a close, return to sensing your physicality, beginning with your feet and toes, then moving up through your legs, hips, abdomen, chest, shoulders, arms, hands, fingers, neck, head, and face. Slowly open your eyes from the deep presence within your body.

Finally, take a Love Breath: inhale deeply with your whole body, then exhale through your mouth with a soft "Hahhhhhhh" sound. Repeat this three times to seal your practice.

∞

PRACTICE EVERY DAY

You'll receive the greatest benefit by practicing this meditation daily. It is best to mediate in the morning, upon waking, before stepping into the activities of the day. This meditation cultivates relaxation, receptivity, and perseverance—the staying power that supports both achieving and maintaining optimal health. These same qualities are also key in developing your capacity to meet the hardships and challenges we all face in our lives. There is not a single situation in life that does not call us to embody ourselves fully—integrating heart, mind, and body—yet most of us remain fragmented and disembodied.

The more you dedicate a set time each day to cultivating awareness in your body—filling up the volume of your body and connecting with the Divine, as we did in the meditation—the more naturally you become embodied, grounded in peace, and less reactive to both outer and inner discord, becoming less a slave to circumstance. The body is endless, so in your meditation, you can include more and more of yourself. Journey into your organs, into your blood vessels, and even into your tiny cells. Work toward experiencing them as pure energy, emptiness, no-thingness.

THE BREATH

The word for "breath" in Persian is "dam," which also means "the moment." Awareness of our breath brings us into the present moment. Many adults take about twenty breaths per minute, yet that this frequency of breathing is not only unnecessary, it can also keep us stuck in a chronic stress response. By breathing in a slow, even rhythm, we create balance in the autonomic nervous system between the sympathetic—the fight-or-flight response—and the parasympathetic—the relaxation response. Inhalation activates the sympathetic system, while exhalation, as the relaxation phase of the breath, engages the parasympathetic system. This shift slows brainwaves and heart rate, lowers blood pressure, and elicits inner calm and relaxation.

The pause after exhalation allows carbon dioxide to gently build in the blood, enhancing the vagus nerve's calming effect on the heart and further stimulating the parasympathetic system. This brings a profound sense of ease to both mind and body. In this pause, we touch the the still point where inner clarity and spiritual insight can arise—what is seen in many mystical traditions as a doorway to the eternal now.

You need to activate your diaphragm, the primary muscle of breathing, which contracts and moves downward into your abdominal cavity as you inhale. This creates negative pressure in the chest cavity, allowing air to flow in through your nostrils and fill the empty space. If it helps, place your hands on your lower ribs and feel them expand outward as you breathe in and soften toward the midline as you exhale.

Breathing through your nose allows for a 10 percent greater oxygen uptake into your lungs. The nose also conditions the air you take in by warming, humidifying, and purifying it before sending it through the respiratory canal. It also continuously releases nasal nitric oxide that helps sterilize the air. Mouth breathing does not do this, as it lacks a filtration system.

Generally speaking, your mouth is for eating and your nose is for breathing. You can, of course, breathe through your mouth, but it is actually a backup system for breathing. Most species in the wild—unless stressed or sick, breathe through their nose. Humans, however, are unusual in that many develop a pattern of chronic mouth breathing even while at rest. This habit can trap the body in sympathetic dominance, with symptoms such as anxiety, muscle pain, poor sleep, poor digestion, weight gain, and a compromised immune system. It can also alter facial structure: the face narrowing and elongating, the oral cavity shrinking, and the jaw retracting—changes that can lead to crowded teeth, narrower airways, and smaller sinuses. Naturally, we breathe through our mouth when we eat, speak, laugh, sigh, and yawn, and there are some exercises and breathing techniques that emphasize exhaling through the mouth to release tension and pent-up emotions. Even so, nasal breathing is the foundation for healthy, balanced respiration.

The Love Breath

In Rumi's *Masnavi-ye Ma'navi*, I once read: "There is a type of breathing that is constriction and there is another that opens you to infinity."[4] I call the second type of breathing the Love Breath. With it, you inhale with your whole body and exhale with a long, pleasurable "Hahhhhhhh"— just as I guided you to do toward the end of our meditation.

When I taught the Love Breath in one of my workshops years ago, a student said, "Oh, I just took a whole weekend workshop on this type of breathing. It is called the Oxytocin Breath." What she was referring to is the stimulation of the vagus nerve that occurs when we take a deep breath in and release with a resonant "Hahhhhhhh." The vagus nerve—the primary bridge between our brain and body—connects to nearly all our major organs (except the adrenals and thyroid). Through the Love Breath, the vagus nerve helps trigger the release of oxytocin, often called the hormone of love and connection.

Oxytocin eases anxiety, fosters relaxation, builds trust, and supports psychological stability. Not surprisingly, research shows, "high levels of this 'love hormone' in couples during the first six months of a relationship."[5] Oxytocin has an anti-anxiety effect, which induces relaxation, a sense of trust, and psychological stability. Because it is released in lovemaking and regulates both childbirth and lactation, oxytocin is also known as "the great facilitator of life."[6]

The Love Breath literally makes you feel like you are in love. It relaxes you and radiates ease outward, soothing those around you. You can use it whenever you feel anxious, nervous, or burdened by bad news—when you're in an argument with someone, or about to react to something unpleasant. You can also use it when you feel joyful or inspired, as well as while you dance. All of these states activate the vagus nerve in ways similar to the Love Breath.

A highly activated, well-functioning vagus nerve supports profound physical, mental, and emotional benefits: lowering the risk of heart disease, enhancing gut motility, regulating blood pressure and glucose balance, aiding fat metabolism, reducing inflammation, improving fertility, and easing anxiety and depression. Even more, the vagus nerve shapes how we connect with one another—it links to the nerves that regulate emotional expression, eye contact, and our ability to attune to human speech. The vitality of the vagus nerve is woven into our capacity for deep connection and our natural impulse toward generosity.

SILENCE

Silence is the sacred ground from which presence arises, allowing us to still our mind, relax our body, connect with our soul, and attune to the living pulse of the Earth. You need silence to listen to the voice of guidance streaming from the Beloved through all and everything. Silence brings you into yourself and into communion with the Beloved and all of existence. You need silence to tune into the greater music and to be one of the instruments participating harmoniously as a member of the greater orchestra of life.

But a great many of us don't create music. Instead, we make noise. To create music, we must become quiet enough to hear the sounds around us—the natural sounds, the music of the Earth, of the universe. Yet all too often, we are busy making noise with our machinery and our loud talking—so much so that we are no longer able to listen. With our noise, we are disruptive to ourselves, to the Earth and her community of beings, and to the universe. Just imagine this noisy planet of ours orbiting through the solar system, accompanied by the constant clamor of traffic, planes, leaf blowers, chainsaws, bombs, blaring TVs and radios, and so on.

We need to disrupt our disruptiveness, which has become our norm. We all need to intentionally lower our noise levels—both the machinery we use and our own voices. I am often amazed at how much incessant talking fills holy places: a beautiful beach in Kauai, a windy trail through the breathtaking Sierras, or shrines such as Hagia Sophia, Chartres Cathedral, or Rumi's mausoleum. We travel for many hours and invest much to reach these places, yet we fill them with our own chatter instead of becoming empty enough to receive something new, something unknown. As "tourists," we forget that we are at once guests in a foreign culture and stewards of our home, the Earth, everywhere we go. Let us remember that our conduct needs to be infused with adab—soul courtesy.

I must also admit that sometimes I may be outwardly silent, yet inwardly my mind is filled with incessant chatter. Our noise dominates the environment. Imagine how all living beings must feel about it. Most likely, they tune us out, just as we tune out the din of our surroundings to stay sane. But all that tuning out consumes energy. Wouldn't it be much better if we used our energy to minimize our noise levels and to truly listen—for the benefit of the world and ourselves?

We need silence in order to listen for and receive guidance. This is the essence of Sama. Noise prevents us from turning inward to receive the wisdom that can make us whole and live on a soul level in the material world.

Silent Fast One Day a Week

I invite you to hold silence for one full day each week. For that day, minimize your noise pollution: refrain from speaking unnecessarily and avoid anything that makes excessive noise, including television and radio. If possible, don't drive a car or motorcycle unless it is hybrid or electric. By practicing silence in this way, we can begin to counter the catastrophic levels of noise pollution—and attune more deeply to who we truly are and why we are here.

EXPLORE RESISTANCE

You can be fully in your body, regardless of physical constraints. It is important to uncover areas in your body where there is resistance to embodiment. Often discomfort, pain, or disease will make us avoid being present. You need to be steadfast and inquire into why this resistance is there—not only with your mind, but also from a visceral sense in your body. Don't avoid the hard yet rewarding work of sincere inquiry. Don't take the shortcut of denial or try to transcend what is there. This only prolongs the process of true embodiment. Your pain, discomfort, and disease are gateways into becoming whole. They cannot be bypassed.

Resistance often arises from past trauma, physical illness, or ingrained protective mechanisms that once helped you survive but now limit you. To explore this resistance, begin by gently noticing where in your body you feel tension, numbness, or avoidance. Ask yourself: "What does this sensation need?" Instead of trying to force openness, approach these areas with curiosity and care. The more you inquire into them with compassion from an embodied place—sensing the living Earth beneath you, releasing your weight into her, and allowing the energy of the One to move through you—the more likely these resistances are to soften and resolve. As we progress in our journey together, we will explore how to identify areas of resistance and work with and through them.

If you have a history of trauma, chronic illness, or pain, resistance may feel overwhelming or even unsafe to approach. It is important to go slowly, with a strong sense of choice and agency. Simply placing your hand on the resistant area and breathing into it can be a powerful first step. If your resistance is too intense, seeking a supportive guide—a therapist, healer, or teacher—can provide a safe container for deeper exploration. The goal is to fill up the volume of your body with awareness and simultaneously experience yourself as pure energy, pure awareness. To truly *be*, you also need to *not be*—to let go of attachment to your physical form. Since we are more energy than matter, the less we identify with the material aspects of ourselves—our body, personality, possessions, and the known—the more we open to our true nature which is energy, interconnected with all that is. From this awareness, our experience of living in a body and in the physical world shifts dramatically. We begin to experience ourselves as souls in this world, taking things less personally and holding a broader perspective on life and events.

BODY INQUIRY
with audio component

I invite you to reflect on your relationship with your body through the following questions:

> How do you feel about your body?

> To what extent is your attitude toward your body a belief you have inherited from your family, your culture, or your community? How does this differ from how *you* genuinely feel about your body?

> What do you tell yourself about your body? Do you say things like, "I'm fat, I'm short, I'm ugly, my hands are too big, my calves are too chunky, my toes are weird, etc."? If so, who in you says this? Would you speak this way about a temple or a natural sanctuary that you deeply admire and cherish?

Shine a light on your relationship with your body, this holiest of holy temples. If your relationship with your body feels broken or strained, reframe it with compassion and re-establish it on a new foundation. Remember, whatever you plant will grow and blossom. Plant the seed of kindness and respect toward your body and witness what unfolds.

∞

Remember, presence is the foundation of embodiment. It begins in your body—in the deep awareness of your breath, your sensation, and your connection to the Earth. Let it transform how you inhabit your body and your life.

I recommend keeping a journal of your reflections after each practice, noting sensations, insights, or shifts you experience. Writing anchors your awareness, deepens integration, and helps you witness your own unfolding over time.

5

FREE WILL

What Do You Serve?

We are always channeling something—whether by conscious choice or unconscious habit. We channel our life's purpose. We broadcast our thoughts and beliefs through every action: how we walk, how we speak, what we say, and what we do. This is why it is vital to become aware of the second ray of Dance of Oneness: "you are a channel." Equally important is attuning to what you truly believe in and to the deeper purpose of your life.

Ray 2: You Are a Channel

To fully embody yourself and activate light in your body—becoming living love—you need to awaken and liberate the energy that flows along your central column, the vertical pathway that runs from the crown of your head to your perineum (see Figures 1 and 2). Rumi likens the human body to a ney (reed flute), "with two mouths—one hidden in the lips of the Beloved."[1] In Dance of Oneness, clearing your ney is essential, enabling the light waves of divine music to flow through and be expressed by you.

Understanding the Upward and Downward Spirals

Unlike many physical practices that only emphasize the upward rising of energy along the central channel, in Dance of Oneness both the ascent

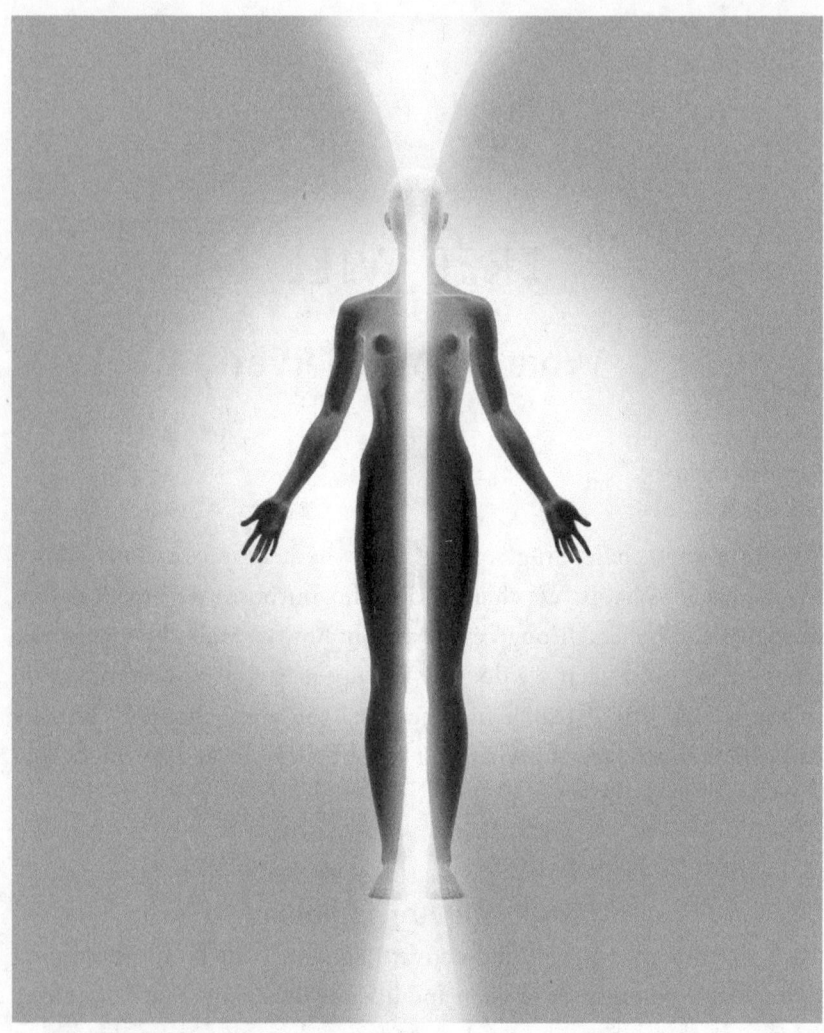

FIGURE 1. The frontal view of the central channel or pathway of the body

and the descent are equally important. The upward spiral is matter—
the feminine, or yin, energy—ascending to meet spirit—the masculine,
or yang, energy. The downward spiral is that of spirit descending and
penetrating matter. They unite in a marriage in the heart. The upward
spiral is about becoming fully human, and the downward spiral is about
activating light in the body and becoming a living embodiment of love.

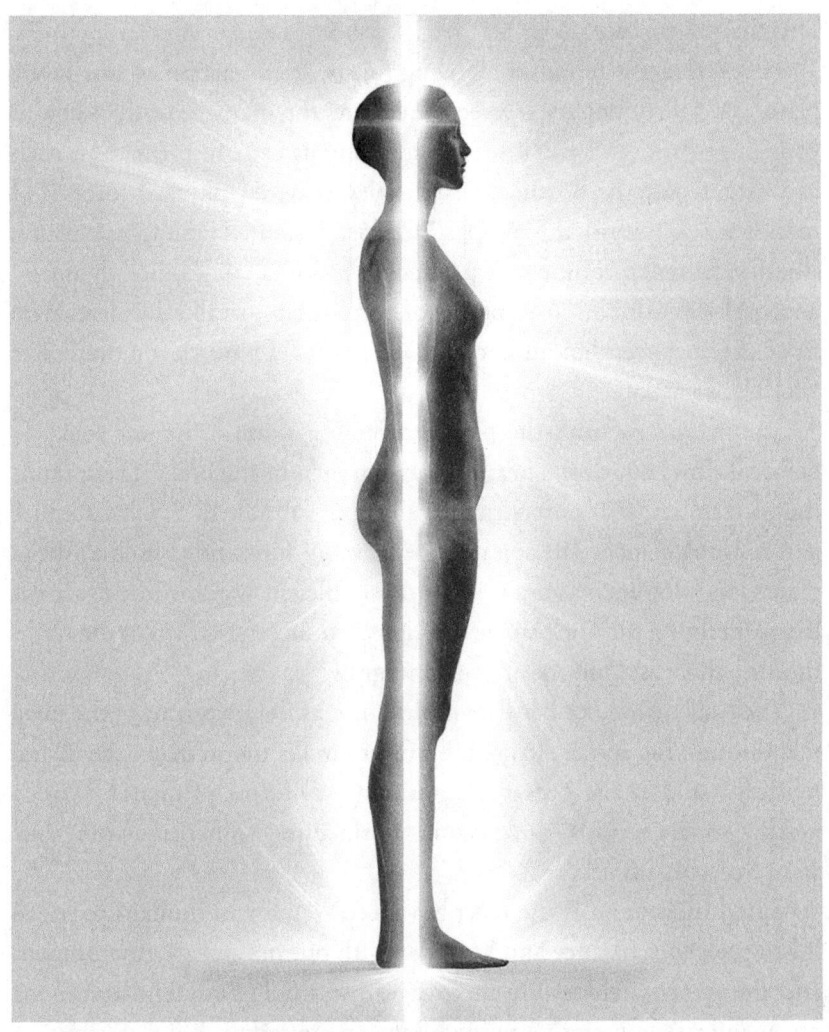

FIGURE 2. The central channel or pathway of the body in silhouette

It is crucial that we create balance and harmony between the body's ascending and descending functions, for these movements reflect the very laws that govern our bodies. If our descending functions become impaired, we will not be able to walk, urinate, defecate, menstruate, or have orgasms—among other essential descending functions.

The Spiral of Life

The spiral shape is found in all living forms, from galaxies to our DNA. Nature is full of spirals at every scale and for many reasons. Look at your fingerprint and you'll see a spiral. Spirals exist in formations such as weather patterns because the interplay between physical forces and matter tends toward this shape. Physicist Nassim Haramein explains: "The fundamental torque that produces the spiral comes directly out of changes in density in the structure of space itself, just like a little change in density between hot air and cold air produces a hurricane that looks a lot like a galaxy."[2]

The heart structures the blood through a spiral in its left ventricle before it flows out of the heart to carry oxygen to the body. The spiral is the pattern nature uses to structure physical substances, resolve conflict, and restore balance. The spiral shape exists in formations such as shells, plants, and flowers because it is the most efficient way for them to grow. By maintaining the same shape through each successive turn of the spiral, they use the least amount of energy to grow.

The Kabbalah describes the visible world as flowering out of the invisible through the spiral. At the innermost level is the source—the divine mystery—and at the outermost, the physical forms of matter. Worlds nesting within worlds, dimensions within dimensions, emanating outward from the unseen.

Spiral movement is the most advanced way for us humans to move. It brings us into balance and harmony with our immediate environment and the greater field of life. It engages the whole body and summons our many strengths into a unified flow. To embody it fully, we must be rooted, centered, flexible, agile, and light.

The Labyrinth

The labyrinth is a spinning spiral. As you enter, you turn and turn in one direction until you arrive at the center—your innermost core, the source—echoing the vision of the Kabbalists. When you leave the center in order to exit, you turn in the opposite direction. In the labyrinth, many dimensions can be accessed simultaneously—past, present, and future. A portal opens through which cosmic energies can be directed to the Earth for healing and regeneration. Spinning or whirling in this sacred shape, which is itself spinning, can open this portal and allow one to become a luminous channel of love in a "Vertical Infinity Axis," which extends from infinitely above to infinitely below. Through conscious intention, this channel can direct healing to specific places and conditions.

Ray 3: Journey in the Upward Spiral to Become Conscious

The journey in the upward spiral of energy along the ney of your body is about coming to know yourself and becoming conscious. By embodying the chakras, or energy centers, along the central column of your body—physically, emotionally, and mentally—you move toward wholeness and become available for a finer energy to descend into you. "Chakra" is a Sanskrit word that literally translates as "wheel," because the life force moving within you spins and rotates. This spinning energy has seven centers in your body, beginning at the base of your spine, rising through your torso, and continuing up to the crown of your head and beyond to the chakra above your head. Chakras 1–3 are the Chakras of Matter; chakras 5–7 are the Chakras of Spirit; and chakra 4, the Heart, connects the two. Chakra 8, located above the head, is your North Star, your energetic portal to higher awareness.

In Dance of Oneness, there are specific practices—dances, exercises, and teachings—designed specifically to activate and balance each of the chakras in the upward spiral. As you will see, most of the Dance of Oneness rays align with specific chakras.

When you activate, open, balance, and embody the teaching of each chakra—and integrate them together in the upward spiral—you become ready to receive the radiance of your soul through the downward spiral. The upward spiral is about coming to know your vessel—your house of body, mind, and emotions—and clearing away the debris of sleep, absence, and forgetfulness. In this spaciousness, your soul can descend through the downward spiral to dwell in its temple, guiding your life and allowing you to become a living embodiment of love.

The following is a brief summary of the chakras (see Figure 3). We will explore them more in depth through the thirteen rays of Dance of Oneness and the practices associated with each ray.

The Chakras of Matter: 1, 2, and 3

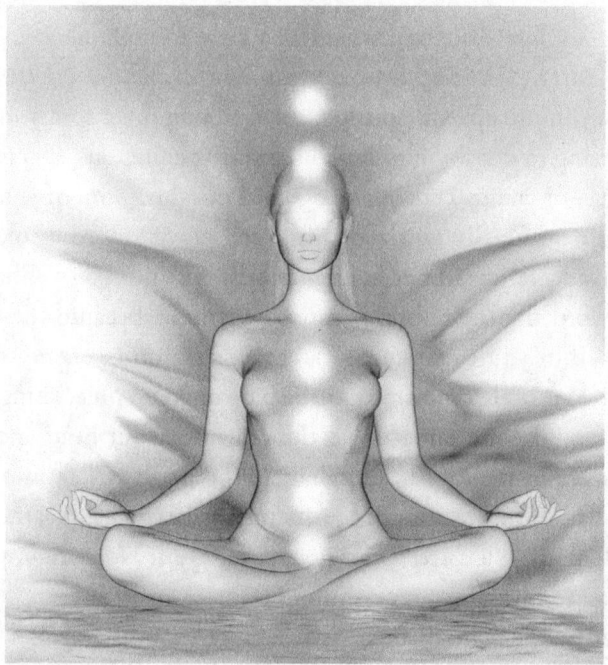

FIGURE 3. The 8 Chakras

1. **Root Chakra**: Located at the base of the spine, Chakra 1 is the center of stability, security, and your basic needs. The areas of influence of this chakra are the perineum, legs, feet, and the immune system. When open and balanced, it fosters a sense of belonging and stability, allowing you to feel safe, fearless and supported. When blocked or closed, it may manifest as low back pain or issues in the hips, knees, ankles, or feet.

Emotionally, you might feel ungrounded, disconnected, or beset by fears of survival and abandonment.

Through meditation, you will learn to ground yourself in the present moment and connect deeply with the Earth, drawing on her stability, security, and strength as the foundation of your body and being.

2. **Sacral Chakra**: Located in the lower abdomen, about two inches below the navel and two inches deep, Chakra 2 is the center of creativity and sexuality. Areas of influence include the pelvis, hips, genitals, sexual organs, and kidneys. When open and balanced, it nurtures a healthy sense of sexuality, and your creativity flows freely. When closed, it may manifest as challenges in the reproductive or urinary systems, or as low back pain. Emotionally, you may struggle with shame, guilt, or blame around sexuality, and carry fears of losing control or being controlled by others.

    Instead of repressing, denying, or allowing your sexual energy to be exploited, recognize it as your sacred creative energy. Through dance, you will ignite this eros and awaken the twin flames of feminine and masculine within, letting them intertwine as a living double helix that sets your whole being ablaze with exuberance.

3. **Solar Plexus Chakra**: Located in the abdomen, extending from the lower belly to the solar plexus or breast bone, Chakra 3 is the center of self. Areas of influence include the entire abdominal cavity, the digestive organs, liver, and gallbladder. When open and balanced, you have a healthy sense of self that is not dependent on what others think of you. When closed, it may manifest as a digestive issues, fear of rejection and criticism, or concerns about physical appearance.

    Through moving with awareness, you will discover that all movement needs to emanate from this center, and by doing so, you come into deeper contact with yourself and cultivate its power. Movement bridges your inner world with the outer, and when you move from the inside out—with a sense of yourself—you begin to feel that you are truly residing within, rather than remaining outwardly focused, as so many of us tend to be.

We will explore how flamenco dance brings balance to the Chakras of Matter. With its emphasis on groundedness, strength, and confidence, this fiery form prepares us to "be here now"—embodying ourselves boldly and shamelessly, facing life exactly as it is.

We will also engage with Tai Chi, a fluid form that can balance the Chakras of Matter by harmonizing our two polar aspects: yin—feminine, receptive, intuitive, life-giving—and yang—masculine, active, intellectual. Through Tai Chi, these energies meet in balance and flow.

Finally, we will turn to the Gurdjieff Work, which invites us to question the habitual ways we think of ourselves by observing from a more objective place. By bringing awareness to our automatic patterns, it helps refine the Chakras of Matter, creating a stable foundation for the upward spiral of energy and the possibility of real transformation.

The Chakra of Union: 4

4. **Heart Chakra**: Located in the center of the chest and midway between the 8 chakras, Chakra 4 unites the lower Chakras of Matter and the upper Chakras of Spirit. It is the gateway through which you connect with others and all of existence—the portal to the quantum field of oneness. Its area of influence extends to the heart and circulatory system, lungs, shoulders, arms, and hands. When open and balanced, it allows love to flow with ease—for yourself and for others. When closed, it may manifest as disharmony in the heart, lungs, or upper body, and may also be felt as guardedness, distrust, or a turning away from your own inner guidance.

   Through a meditative visualization, you will open your heart, petal by petal, like a luminous rose unfolding its light. We will also explore how Persian dance can lead you into the mystery of becoming both lover and beloved of the Beloved, through the ecstasy of adoration.

The Chakras of Spirit: 5, 6, 7, and 8

5. **Throat Chakra**: Located in the throat, Chakra 5 is the center of expression, choice, and willpower. Its influence extends to the neck, throat, thyroid and parathyroid glands, jaw, mouth, and ears. When open and balanced, it supports clear self-expression, truthful speech, and deep listening. When closed, it may manifest as imbalances in the neck, throat, or related glands, or as a constriction in your ability to live and express your authentic self. You may struggle with indecision or, conversely, with controlling tendencies. You may also fall into deception—of yourself or others—and find it difficult to truly listen.

    Through safe, trance-inducing movements, you will learn to release the fear of losing control—a fear that restricts the Throat Chakra—and open into a freer, more authentic expression.

6. **Third Eye Chakra**: Located in the center of the brain and corresponding to the pineal gland, Chakra 6 is the seat of intuition and inner vision—often called the "third eye." It governs the eyes, the brain, the pineal gland, and the neurological system. When open and balanced, it connects you to intuition, imagination, clarity of mind, and visionary insights. When closed, it may manifest as difficulties with the eyes, brain, or nervous system, along with a sense of being cut off from your inner guidance, unable to access your visionary powers or see the larger picture.

    We will connect with this chakra through visualization.

7. **Crown Chakra**: Located on the crown of your head, Chakra 7 is the gateway to spirit, the greater existence, and the eternal—accessible only in the present moment. Its influence

extends to the brain, the nervous system, and the muscular and skeletal systems. When open and balanced, you feel deeply connected with spirit and the greater existence, often experiencing an intimate communion with the Beloved in all that you do. When blocked or closed, you may struggle to perceive realities beyond the physical world, finding it difficult to trust the unseen. Such imbalances can manifest as autoimmune conditions or mysterious ailments that elude medical diagnosis.

Through reflection and inquiry, as well as a walking practice that awakens all the chakras, you will strengthen and embody your connection with spirit.

8. **Soul Star Chakra**: Located just above the head—anywhere from a few inches to three feet—Chakra 8 is your North Star. It serves as the energetic portal to higher awareness, soul-level purpose, and divine guidance. This chakra is the seat of the subconscious mind and interplays with your dream space. In many ways it is similar to the Crown Chakra, yet it is more expansive. Its sphere of influence is the auric field—the luminous energy that surrounds your body.

When activated and balanced, the Soul Star Chakra brings clarity of purpose, illuminating why you are here in this life. With such clarity, you break through limiting beliefs, allowing your authentic self to emerge and guide you with precision. When closed or underactive—when the connection has not yet been made—you may feel lost, without purpose, sluggish, or stuck, yearning without direction. Constant craving can also signal imbalance in this chakra. Emotionally, a closed Charka 8 may manifest as anxiety, cynicism, or depression. You may lack faith—in spirit or in yourself—and even experience ailments that elude medical diagnosis.

You will connect with your Soul Star Chakra through a meditative visualization.

WHAT DO I CHANNEL?
with audio component

I invite you to inquire into what you serve and channel in this present moment.

Sit comfortably, feeling the living Earth beneath your feet, lengthening through your spine. Gently close your eyes, inhale deeply, and as you exhale, allow your whole being to relax into the embrace of the present moment.

Ask yourself, "What do I serve in this moment? What am I choosing to channel?"

Notice any immediate answers that arise—whether care, love, fear, egoistic aims, or something else. Simply observe without judgement.

Stay in the awareness of what you serve. Even the simple act of noticing is transformative. Awareness itself begins to shift your orientation, loosening old habits and opening the possibility of choice. Free will lives in moment-to-moment awareness, where you decide what current to strengthen and what to channel into the world.

∞

Remember, what you serve becomes the current shaping your life and the greater field. Each moment invites you to choose—fear or love, separation or unity. In realizing you are a channel, you awaken the power of free will.

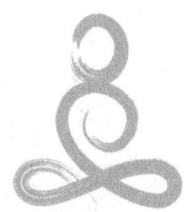

Journey Through Chakras 1–3

Open, Align, and Balance Your Physical Centers

6

EARTHING

Take Root in the Here and Now

Ray 4: Ground Yourself Lovingly in the Earth

Chakra: 1—Muladhara (Root Support)

Location: Base of the spine or coccyx

Anatomical areas of influence: Base of the spine, rectum, legs, feet, and the immune system

Element: Earth

Color: Red

Having entered into presence and gained the awareness that you are a channel for what you believe in, we now move to the fourth ray of Dance of Oneness, which invites you to ground yourself by feeling your energetic roots in the Earth with reverence and gratitude, and to live from this connection. This ray corresponds to the Root Chakra and highlights that one mouth of the channel you are must open downward, connecting you with the Earth. Your health, your well-being, and dance all depend on this living bond with the Earth as Gaia—one of the supreme manifestations of the Divine Mother. The more you revere and honor the Earth, the more alive, vibrant, and radiant you will feel in your body.

Your bond with the Earth is the basis, root, and foundation for all your bonds and relationships. If you don't honor the Earth, you are unable to truly honor your body or your connection with others. More fundamentally, you cannot fully *be*. Most of us live in our heads much of the time and need to actively be reminded that we have a body, that we are connected to the Earth, and that our energy must flow downward as well as upward if we are to embody ourselves fully and live with greater capacity.

In observing people, I have noticed that the habitual tendency is to let our energy rise up. The reason lies in the duality and polarization that have governed our worldview for the past five thousand years. As we already explored, we tend to perceive both mind and spirit as separate from matter and as "superior" in value. Therefore, we tend—often unconsciously—toward a desire to "rise above" what is considered the mire, messiness, and darkness of physicality. In doing so, we unknowingly disembody and fragment ourselves. Patriarchal god-based systems, particularly the Abrahamic religions, directed reverence and prayer upward toward the sky, emphasizing heavenly attainment over embodiment. They condemned the Earth and the body as houses of sin, making it nearly impossible to attain so-called purity or to win the approval of a perfect God in the heavens.

THE EMPHASIS ON "UP"

The overemphasis on ascent and the constant rising of our energy can disturb the body's natural functioning. From the perspective of Chinese medicine, placing too much focus on upward movement can give rise to anger, anxiety, hypertension, ulcers, headaches, and insomnia. It also makes the body stiffer, the muscles tense, and more easily fatigued from being continually engaged. Simply holding ourselves up in this way consumes a great deal of energy.

True suppleness and lightness in the body arise when we release our weight downward, fill the volume of our bodies with loving awareness, and allow ourselves to feel the Earth supporting us—which is to feel the embrace of the Great Mother.

When we live only in our heads rather than inhabiting our whole body, we are more vulnerable to anxiety and nervousness. As magnificent and prolific as our heads may be, the capacity of the tiny, disembodied head is incomparable to the vast capacity we access when the whole body—including the head—is engaged. By simply releasing our weight downward and viscerally attuning to the Earth as a living being, we become happier, more relaxed, and more at home in our own skin. We become more responsive rather than reactive, more present rather than preoccupied, and our pace grows less hurried—yet not necessarily less energized.

All the variations of "high" are generally considered more desirable to those that imply "low," as the English language reveals: superior versus inferior, upper versus lower, elation versus depression, above versus below, ascent versus descent, elevation versus degradation, and the list goes on. But love, the most cherished feeling a human being can experience, is associated with "falling" in the English language—we fall in love.

Where is "up" and where is "down," really? The Earth is constantly rotating, so what is up now will eventually go down, and what is down will rise again—just as the Tao teaches. The Tao, the cyclical relationship of yin and yang, is the symbol of life on Earth: the dance of duality between matter and spirit, body and soul, all contained in the One.

PRACTICE

GROUND IN MOTHER EARTH MEDITATION
with audio component

This meditation is a way of deepening your bond with the living Earth. It is not meant for daily repetition, but rather as a touchstone you can return to whenever you feel scattered, fragmented, or adrift—an invitation to root again in her steady embrace.

Time required: 10–20 minutes

Begin with the Basic Meditation (chapter 4).

Within a global awareness of your whole body, let the soles of your feet awaken to the living Earth if you are seated on a chair, or allow your legs and feet to soften into the Earth if you are sitting cross-legged on the ground.

Visualize yourself sitting on the planet Earth.

Within a global awareness of your body, bring your attention to the base of your spine, your tailbone, and your perineum— the region between your pubic arch and your tailbone. Rest your awareness on the meridian point in the perineum called Huiyin (Meeting of the Yin), located midway between the genitals and the anus. Huiyin is the gateway through which the body receives and absorbs the Earth's yin energy, carried upward through the three yin leg meridians: liver, spleen, and kidney. (See Figure 5 at the start of chapter 8.)

Energetically draw the energy of the Earth slowly up your legs and into your perineum, the base of your spine, your hips, and your buttocks.

Maintain your connection with the energy of the Earth (Earth chi) in the lower, foundational part of your body as you flow with your breath and engage in the following inquiry. Listen sincerely for a response before moving on to the next, as you hold a global awareness of your body. Let the questions and answers arise from this embodied awareness— not just from your head—and remain present in your body as you listen.

Can I just be? If not, what is keeping me from simply being?

Can I simply release my weight into the Earth instead of holding myself up? In what part(s) of my body do I hold myself up?

Can I soften and let go of the holding in those places?

Who, or what, is the Earth for me? How do I feel toward the Earth?

How do I feel about being *here*, in this moment? Can I say I am fully here?

When you have completed your inquiries, take three Love Breaths (chapter 4).

Anchor yourself in your body and in the Earth—Gaia, our living Mother. Allow stability, security, and trust to permeate the foundation of your body—your feet, legs, and base of your spine—as you deepen your connection with the Earth. Stay connected with your breath, inhaling and exhaling slowly from your nose.

Experience your body and the body of the Earth as one—no separation. Let her powerful, loving presence spread gently into your pelvis, your genitals, your lower belly, and your lower back.

Allow this energy to gradually fill your whole abdomen.

Invite Gaia's unconditional love to rise up into your heart and upper back.

Feel yourself held in her embrace, and linger in the silence for as long as you can, listening for any messages or guidance.

When you are ready to close the practice, begin by gently wiggling your toes. Take three Love Breaths.

Sense your feet, legs, hips, abdomen, heart center, neck, and whole head.

Open your eyes from the deep connection with Mother Earth. Drink in her radiance—her generous beauty shining all around you, reflected in everyone you meet, and alive within you.

∞

Awakening the Soles of Your Feet to the Earth

Now that you have entered into a deep connection with Mother Earth, I invite you to let the soles of your feet awaken to the living Earth as you sit, stand, and walk. The doorway to presence is the body infused with loving awareness—this is embodiment. And the doorway into embodiment begins with letting the soles of your feet awaken to the living Earth. Through this simple yet profound act, you claim your place here and now, and begin to make peace with physicality and all that it encompasses.

7

SACRED SEXUALITY

The Dance of Polarity

*Ray 5: Embody Your Sexuality as Your Creative
Life Force in the Sacred Union of Polarities*

Chakra: 2—Svadisthana (Her Special Abode)

Location: Genitals to navel area

Anatomical areas of influence: Sexual organs, genitals,
bladder, hips, lower spine

Element: Water

Color: Orange

Maintaining the loving connection you've established with the Earth,
I invite you to now focus on your sexuality. Human sexuality mirrors
the perpetual act of creation unfolding at every level of life throughout the universe. Your sexuality is your vital life force. It is the seat of
your generative, creative energies. This is where your radiance, the fire
for your movement, and your dance itself needs to be fueled from. Your
sexuality is your vital life force. It is the seat of your generative, creative

energies—the inner flame that lights your radiance, ignites your dance, and continually fuels it.

Instead of repressing, denying, or allowing this energy to be exploited, know that your sexual energy is your creative energy. The energy that gives birth to children is the same one that fuels art, ignites passion, and sustains a creative life. Sexual energy nourishes your aliveness and your magnetism. Without it, both your dance and your life grow flat, lifeless—nearly comatose. As American modern dancer and choreographer Martha Graham said, "So much of the movement comes from a pelvic thrust." She was known to admonish women dancers by saying, "You're simply not moving your vagina, dear!"[1]

WHAT IS SEXUALITY?

Sexuality is raw power—long misunderstood and seldom explored spiritually, except in a few sacred traditions, among them Taoism and Tantra,[2] that honor it as a gateway to higher states of consciousness.

A path that does not revere sexuality as sacred cannot be a true path. It is incomplete within itself and leads to fragmentation in those who follow it. This imbalance is revealed in the countless sex scandals that surface in religious and spiritual communities that repress or attempt to sublimate our vital sexual energy.

The sexual act opens us to ecstasy, the sacred gateway through which the soul communes and unites with the Divine. In this state, the individual self dissolves into the universal self. When sexuality is honored as sacred love-making, it awakens a current of energy that forms a transcendent bond, in which the union of bodies becomes also a union of souls, where the lovers experience themselves as embodied expressions of the Divine. This awakening accelerates their spiritual evolution.

When integrity and love are absent, however, physical union can leave people feeling empty, disconnected, or even burdened by shame—toward themselves or the act itself. This is why it is essential to bring care and awareness to our sexuality, in whatever form we choose to express it.

And here is the good news: for those who are not in a committed relationship and who do not wish to approach sexuality casually, the same current of spiritual energy that is awakened when sexuality is fused with love can also be accessed through dance. Dance, too, can open us to ecstasy, to communion and union with the Divine.

DANCE IS LOVE-MAKING

Dance is a form of love-making—an invitation to continually make love with the present moment, engaging with life sensually.

What is sensuality to you? At the heart of authentic sensuality is the capacity to surrender: to offer yourself fully to what is here, right now; to embrace your body as you are; and to simply be, as nature is. From this surrender arises a joy of being—a quiet enjoyment, a smile from within, a sense of ease and relaxation that can only be accessed in and through the body.

The invitation is to let your dance harmonize the feminine and masculine energies within you, blending your sexual energy with your heart and mind. As these energies fuse, your dance becomes a living flame— emanating vitality, fire, and light from your sexual center. Ultimately, your dance can become a love-making with the Beloved—the union of spirit and matter in your body, expressed in ever-expanding ways: wondrous and sublime, sensual and wild, noble and tender.

THE KIDNEYS, THE ORGANS OF WATER AND FIRE

Our sexual energy is composed of the twin feminine and masculine flames. In Chinese medicine, the kidneys are directly connected to our sexual energy and are said to house these twin flames. In modern science, the kidneys regulate the composition of blood by filtering waste and excess water. In Chinese medicine, however, they are considered the most fundamental organ system, holding the genetic blueprint of our inherent constitution and influencing how healthy and vital we will be.

We have two kidneys and, from the perspective of Chinese medicine, the left kidney carries yin energy while the right carries yang. Even in their shape—echoing the Taoist symbol of yin and yang—the kidneys

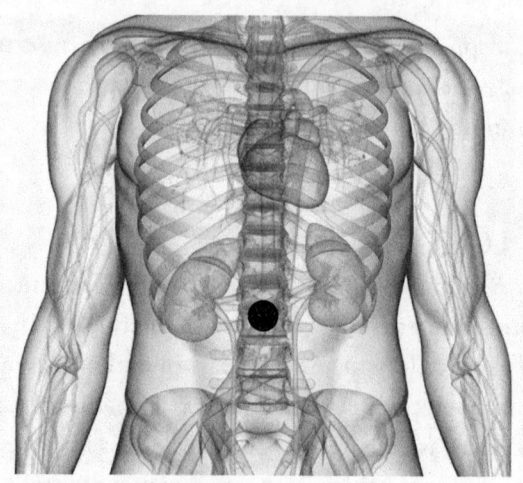

FIGURE 4. Mingmen (Gate of Life) meridian point

are seen as the organs of water and fire, the abode of yin and yang, the sea of essence, and arbiters of life and death. Our growth, development, maturation, sexual vitality, and reproduction are governed by the kidneys. All bodily functions rely on the heat provided by kidney chi (energy) and the meridian point known as Mingmen (Gate of Life).

Located in the spine beneath the second lumbar vertebra, between the kidneys and roughly in line with the navel (see Figure 4), Mingmen is one of the body's most powerful meridian points. It blends the dual energies of kidney yin and yang, strengthens the low back, builds life energy, and increases libido.

Kidney yin and yang form the foundation of our body. They are interconnected and interdependent, and they restrain each other to maintain a balance of yin and yang in the whole body. We would be enlightened if only our psyche would learn to live the balance between the yin and yang energies that are inherent in our body.

FAVORING THE MASCULINE ENERGY

The imbalance and conflict between the masculine and feminine—tilted in favor of the masculine for the last five thousand years—has shaped not only the world we live in, but also our inner world. Isn't it striking that to simply *be* has become something we must learn—or rather unlearn or re-pattern—because it is not our default state? For millennia, the yang, active, masculine energy of "doing" has been elevated above the yin, receptive, feminine energy of "being," to the point that we now have to literally train ourselves to simply *be*.

Most women I've met and taught identify more with their masculine side than their feminine side. They don't honor or value the yin qualities of suppleness, softness, delicate grace, lusciousness, receptivity, and simply being as much as they regard the yang characteristics of doing and achieving tasks and goals. Many also wear an armor around their hips.

THE ARMORS WE WEAR

Most of us, in fact, wear armor—at varying intensities—around our hips, abdomen, chest, and neck as a default way of defending ourselves. Our bodies are overrun and dominated by fear. I first discovered these armors by observing myself. One day, while washing dishes, I noticed I was squeezing my buttocks and holding my hips rigidly. I wondered why I was engaging these parts of my body so intensely while doing something as simple as washing dishes! I consciously relaxed my hips and buttocks and continued, yet after a few moments, I noticed the tightness had returned. My mind had wandered, and with it, my body had tensed up again. Washing dishes doesn't require this much intensity—as if I were preparing for battle (though for some of us, housework can sometimes feel like a battle!).

From then on, I became aware of the armor I wear in different parts of my body, and I began to observe this phenomenon in others. Again and again, I discovered that these armors are almost always the residue of trauma. Our default state, as modern humans, tends toward fear and tightness—toward defense or attack.

Most of us don't know how to protect ourselves energetically with discernment grounded in love and in awareness of what to allow into our field. More than anything, we suffer from ignorance—ignorance of love.

The invitation for the carrier of light is to become the one others can turn to for love. Can we be the ones who, even in conflict, remember that what is most needed is love—and recognize how the traumas we carry can lead us to act in painful ways, calling for the healing balm of love?

The path of living love requires rigor, sincerity, struggle, suffering, and grace—a combination that melts the armors in your body. Self-acceptance is the key. The first step is to come home to yourself and notice what the home turf is like. Is it in disarray? Are your hips—or another part of your body—out of balance? Do you hold one hip higher than the other? You can't just say, "I'll keep walking around like this, and it will hopefully get better one day." You need to shift your perception and heal—or seek help. Explore acupuncture, therapy, or other forms of support if you don't know how to heal yourself. Pay attention to the practical, physical signs, because they reveal where your shadow resides and where your potential lies.

HIP ARMOR

Shame is the root cause of the armor around our hips. It arises not only from our personal sexual wounds, but also from the collective stigma and degradation of human sexuality that have accumulated over the last five thousand years. Yet sexuality was not always stigmatized. In ancient cultures, it was often celebrated as a sacred and natural part of life, intimately connected with creation, fertility, and the Divine. Only through the gradual shifts in societal, religious, and cultural beliefs did sexuality become entangled with shame, guilt, and suppression.

In Goddess-centered cultures, sexuality was honored and freely expressed, revered as a natural and sacred current of life. One of the names of the Sumerian Goddess Inanna was "Opener of the Womb," and her priestesses served her by initiating people into sacred sexuality. In a similar spirit, the Tantric traditions teach that sexuality is holy and meant to be sanctified.

When we notice tension in our hips, it is important to pause and and ask: "What is the source of this tension?" In the absence of personal sexual trauma, the tension often carries the memory of ancestral wounds around sexuality. Our body remembers what our ancestors endured. Aware that collective ideologies have long distorted the way we approach our sexuality, we are called to look inward and discern how these beliefs live in us. Where do we still uphold patriarchal views—for example, those that cast the feminine as inferior, sinful, manipulative, a temptress or deceiver? To recognize this conditioning within ourselves is to begin the sacred work of healing.

ADAM AND EVE

Take the myth of Adam and Eve as an example. In its common interpretation, Eve is demonized and blamed as the source of sin and humanity's suffering. But from another perspective, Eve, as the receptive principal of existence, offers wisdom—symbolized by the apple—to Adam, who represents the active principal. The receptive is the source of guidance and wisdom from which the active is called to take direction.

By giving Adam the apple, Eve offers him the wisdom of both shadow and light, essentially saying, "Eat this apple and live in your body!" Living in a body comes with immense challenges, both profound and endless. Therefore, it is crucial to explore what restricts us physically—such as tension in our hips—and understand why and where it originates.

We need to ask how collective stories and myths manifest in our lives and begin to replace shame with acceptance, compassion, and honor. If you've ever felt degraded or shamed, it is important to acknowledge and understand that experience. When it feels safe and supportive, speaking your truth—whether directly to the person who shamed you, or in another healing context—can help release the burden you've been carrying. From this place, you can begin to extend compassion to yourself, and, when you are ready, perhaps even to the other, recognizing that on some level, they didn't know any better. As Yeshua said, "Forgive them, for they know not what they do."[3]

UNITE, INTEGRATE, AND BALANCE POLARITIES

In the Sacral Chakra, the unified energy of the Root Chakra and its sacred teaching that "all is one" becomes divided into polarities: feminine/masculine, yin/yang, sun/moon, negative/positive, and so on. Understanding the relationship of these opposites and bringing them into balance is intrinsic to the fifth ray of Dance of Oneness and the key to opening and activating this chakra.

What we see as opposites are more interdependent than we imagine. This secret is revealed in the symbol of the Tao—the yin/yang, the cyclical relationship of light and dark that alternate, not as enemies but as utterly inseparable complements. This symbol shows how the universe is a perpetual dance of polarities rising up, connecting through a third force, and returning to the mystery in a constantly attuned and adjusted balance.

When we only cultivate or insist on one side, we become unbalanced and unhealthy. Yin is the feminine energy—being, calmness, mystery, darkness. Yang is the masculine energy—doing, activity, exuberance, the light. The entire phenomenal universe exists because of the tension between opposites. Birth and death, growth and decay, gain and loss, success and failure, hot and cold are a few. Polarities are part of existence and, of course, every relationship. And boy, do we live in a polarized world today.

We cannot eliminate polarities on the physical level, but we can reconcile, harmonize, and blend them through surrender and acceptance. Whenever we accept what is, something deeper emerges. Even in hatred, when we accept what we feel without running away, we begin to transform it. It may still be present, but suddenly we are in a vaster place where it no longer has the same charge. This is why feeling and expressing our emotions are so important. As Rumi says, "Learn the alchemy true human beings know. The moment you accept what troubles you've been given, the door will open . . . because what hurts you blesses you . . ."[4]

Without opposites interacting, there is no dance—up and down, side to side, stillness and motion, contraction and expansion, flexion and extension. In dance, opposites harmonize yet remain distinct. In Dance of Oneness, we cultivate both the feminine qualities of softness, fluidity, and sensuality as well as the masculine qualities of strength, speed, and determination.

SACRED SENSUALITY

My vision of sacred sensuality was formed through my confrontation with two major shadows: the repression of the feminine in much of Islamic practice and the degradation of the feminine across Western media. Both, in different ways, have profoundly distorted our relationship to the feminine. I'll share an example of just how deeply this repression runs.

A woman came to one of my workshops in Turkey called *Body of Light*. On the first day she introduced herself as a professional belly dancer and a Naqshbandi Sufi, which has traditionally been one of the more conservative Tarighats (Orders). She shared that in her life, being a belly dancer and a conservative Sufi had always felt distinct. She chose to study with me because she felt I had integrated the sacred with the sensual.

So we began, and she resisted me at every step. To her, some of what I guided the group into felt blasphemous. In the end, she decided the two sides needed to stay separate—a split I have witnessed in many Muslim women. Some do not wear the hijab in daily life but put it on to pray, and this has always perplexed me. Why must communing with the Divine require veiling? Why not offer all of ourselves to the Divine and be intimate with the Beloved without reservation? Who are we worshipping when we feel compelled to hide parts of ourselves—the punishing father in the sky? This father, we are told, demands that women veil themselves and walk behind their husbands rather than beside them, and disapproves of belly dancing. Why do we continue to carry such painful divisions within ourselves?

I feel a similar pain when I witness the degradation of the feminine in much of Western popular media. I believe everyone should be free to explore their body and express themselves as they wish, but when that expression is shared with billions of impressionable young people, the message carries responsibility. Too often, pop stars with massive followings exploit their bodies and sexuality in ways that degrade rather than uplift, in pursuit of money and fame. What kind of role model does this create? To me, this is not empowerment but manipulation—sexuality used for power rather than for love. True empowerment arises from authenticity, from being at ease in one's own skin and inspiring others to feel the same about themselves.

Women who use sexuality for manipulation reinforce patriarchal clichés of the feminine as untrustworthy and feed reactionary misogyny. The oppression and the exploitation of the feminine are two sides of the same coin, branches of the same root. Both stem from confusion about the true nature of the feminine: mother, who nourishes and births life, and mystery, the unfathomable depth from which all arises. At the root of this confusion lies the unhealed conflict between the masculine and the feminine. Instead of harmonizing with the receptive, the active seeks to dominate it.

PRACTICE

REFLECT ON YOUR FEMININE AND MASCULINE ENERGIES
with audio component

I invite you to pause and reflect on your feminine and masculine energies and ask yourself the following question:

> In my daily life, do I feel there is a balance between my feminine (being) and masculine (doing) sides? Do I spend as much time nurturing myself and attending to my body and soul with rest, meditation, sacred dance, and conscious movement as I do to accomplishing tasks and goals?

∞

INFINITY WAVES—MARRYING THE TWIN FLAMES

with video component

This practice invites you to harmonize your feminine and masculine energies, weaving them into a vital union in your body.

Time Required: 5-15 minutes

Stand with your feet shoulder-width apart, parallel to each other. Release your tailbone downward. Soften your knees. Flow with your breath, and come into touch with your ney (reed flute).

We will start with the backward-moving Infinity Wave, as if drawing a horizontal "8" on the ground with your tailbone moving side to side (like the infinity sign).

Keeping your feet rooted in the ground, begin with the left hip moving to the back. Circle your hips counterclockwise to the left, tracing one of the circles of the "8" on the ground with your tailbone by flowing into your left hip. Continue to complete the "8" by circling your hips in a clockwise circle to the right, flowing into your right hip. Continue flowing from one side to the other.

Do twenty sets. Fill up the volume of your hips. Rest your hands on your pelvic bones if you wish, guiding the current of the wave.

Once you feel comfortable with the movement, begin to visualize your twin flames—your feminine/yin side on the left, and your masculine/yang side on the right—meeting in the eternal dance.

Stay in touch with your ney where the two flames meet, holding the intention of union. Let them spiral toward one another, merge in harmony, and become one flame at the center.

As you grow more fluid, let the Infinity Wave rise upward: through your abdomen, heart center, shoulders and arms, neck and throat, and finally your head—until your entire body flows in the Infinity Wave.

To bring the backward-moving Infinity Wave to a close, release with a playful shaking of the hips, twisting your waist side to side vigorously in delight.

Repeat the entire sequence with the forward-moving Infinity Wave: now let your left hip move forward and circle clockwise to the right. Then lead with your right hip and circle counter clockwise to the left. Repeat this twenty times.

Visualize the feminine and masculine flames dancing together and merging as one in the center—in your ney.

If you feel ready, allow the backward moving Infinity Wave to rise upward: through your abdomen, heart center, shoulders and arms, neck and throat, and finally your head—until your entire body flows in a sacred Infinity Wave.

To bring the forward-moving Infinity Wave to a close, shake your hips once more, twisting your waist side to side, loosening everything with joyful abandon.

Come to stillness. Stand for a minute or so, sensing the union of feminine and masculine energies alive within you. Notice how you feel. Which Infinity Wave felt more natural and intuitive to you? When you are ready to close the practice, take a Love Breath.

∞

Your sexuality has the potential to open you to the Divine through ecstasy and bliss. When shared with another, this potential is magnified through love, emotional resonance, and spiritual compatibility. An anonymous thirteenth-century Kabbalist wrote in the *Iggeret ha-Qodesh*,

> When sexual union is for the sake of heaven, there is nothing as holy or pure . . . thereby, one becomes partner with God in the act of creation. This is the secret meaning of the saying of the sages . . . when two beings, devoted to each other in heart, mind, and body, unite, the divine presence is between them.[5]

It is essential to integrate your sexual energy with your heart and mind in order to become whole and sovereign in your sexuality. As you cultivate intimacy—a loving, kind attitude—toward yourself, and build a strong container for these three energies (sexuality, heart, and mind), you become more able to dissolve the armor of shame around your hips and open to to sharing love in a sexual-spiritual union with another.

8

THE INNER SUN

Opening to Your Sovereignty

*Ray 6: Love Who You Are, Allowing Movement
to Emanate from Your Center*

Chakra: 3—Manipura (City of the Shining Jewel)

Location: Extends from lower abdomen to breast bone or solar plexus

Anatomical areas of influence: Entire abdominal cavity, including all the organs; middle spine

Element: Fire

Color: Yellow

Rooted in the Earth and honoring your sexuality as a sacred union of polarities, you are now ready to meet yourself anew through the sixth ray of Dance of Oneness. This ray invites you to find your center and to let all movement arise from it and return to it. Consider this "center" as the home of the self, which in yogic anatomy corresponds to Chakra 3. In Taoist energetic anatomy, it is known as the lower Dantian.

The Taoist sages identified three Dantians, or "energy centers," in the body that store and radiate energy, much like a battery. The upper Dantian is located in the head, the middle in the chest, and the lower in the abdomen. The lower Dantian is the most emphasized in Taoist training, as it is the foundation where martial artists and meditators are first taught to focus their concentration. It is regarded as the wellspring of physical strength and the source of stamina.

Energetically, the lower Dantian bridges Chakras 2 and 3. Its physical location corresponds to Chakra 2, but its field of energy encompasses Chakra 3. The lower Dantian lies at the center of a triangle formed by drawing lines between the navel, the Mingmen point on the spine, and the Huiyin point in the perineum (see Figure 5). Viewed three-dimensionally, the points of the navel, Mingmen, and Huiyin form a downward-facing energy cone. This configuration allows the lower Dantian to draw chi

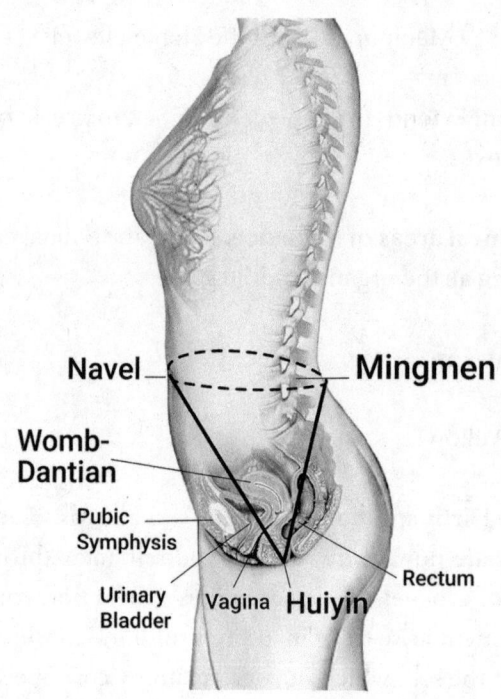

FIGURE 5. The location of the Womb-Dantian

from the Earth through Huiyin and transform it into heat and vital energy for the body. It also acts as a reservoir where heat and energy are stored. In the female body, the lower Dantian corresponds to the uterus, which is why I call this center the Womb-Dantian.

In Dance of Oneness, as in Tai Chi and Qigong, you learn to focus and gather your attention in this part of your body, initiating movement from here while staying connected to the Earth. You begin to realize that every movement also needs to return to your Womb-Dantian in a cyclical pattern. This circular movement expands your capacity for energy, strength, and vitality. Through this rhythm, you learn to conserve and generate energy even as you expend it. Exertion no longer drains you; it becomes effortless and invigorating, as you discover how to move with economy and balance. Envision the rotating yin/yang symbol of the Tao in your Womb-Dantian. The initiation of movement from the Womb-Dantian is yang in nature, while the conscious return to the womb-dantian is yin. This cycle conserves, nourishes, and balances your energy.

As you may recall from chapter 3, the word for "womb" in Arabic is "rahm," and in Aramaic, "rahme." Both mean "mercy" and "compassion." In Aramaic, "rahme" is more specifically defined as "an inner motion extending from the center or depths of the body, radiating heat and ardor."[1] This echoes the Taoist description of the lower Dantian as the body's generator of electricity, the source of all energy pathways.

Taoists considered the navel the Earth or root of the body. Taoist master Mantak Chia affirms, "The navel is the origin of energy: from the fertilized ovum the fetus is developed, linked to life by the umbilical cord. After birth the surrounding [outside] energy continues to enter through the same area."[2]

The beatitude attributed to Yeshua from his Sermon on the Mount— "Blessed are those who from their inner wombs birth compassion and mercy, they shall feel its warm arms embracing them back."[3]—not only implies that both women and men have "inner wombs," but it also describes the cyclical current of energy as it arises and returns to the womb. Yeshua was specifically characterizing this current as the birthing and expansion of compassion, a living power that naturally causes one to feel warm, supported, and abundant in return. The true power and source of stamina in your center is compassion itself. The more you act with compassion, the more its warmth and vitality flow back into you. After all, what we give is what we receive.

The invitation, then, is to let compassion flow outward and inward. In Dance of Oneness, even Sama—the sacred whirling—begins with embracing yourself. Only through loving yourself can you awaken to the mystery of being the Beloved's beloved.

To embody this, we keep the outer layer of the abdomen—the rectus abdominis and external obliques—toned yet relaxed, so we can access the true power of kindness and compassion in our Womb-Dantian. This contrasts sharply with the glorification of "hard abs" in contemporary Western culture, which mistakes rigidity for strength and in fact robs us of authentic power. We become followers and sheep-like instead of sovereign lions.

Most of us wear an abdominal armor known as "hard abs" and "suck your belly in." This armor keeps us from being in our center with ease, from accessing our true power, from cultivating an authentic sense of self, and from experiencing a sense of belonging in our body. Through the phenomenon of "hard abs" and "suck your belly in," we are cut off from accessing and embodying ourselves fully. At times, we may even want to avoid feeling ourselves completely, because we may feel unworthy and unable to hold ourselves in high esteem or with love. The impetus for being critical or "hard" on ourselves can also result in "hard abs" and armor. These two dynamics—self-criticism and physical hardening—are so tightly interwoven that it is often hard to discern which comes first.

Either way, the abdominal armor makes us relate to ourselves and our body from the outside, through the lens of what society accepts as the "norm." Many of us may be sucking in our bellies to appear skinny, creating a convincing illusion. Yet in doing so, our true power source grows thin and depleted, for we give it away—allowing ourselves to be lured by outside forces: the media serving a capitalist agenda and its dictates of beauty, or the expectations of culture, family, friends, spouses, and lovers. In this state, our movements no longer arise from our center—because we have lost touch with it—and we remain disconnected from our potential, our self-esteem wavering and dependent on outside approval.

The abdominal armor also interferes with the functioning of our digestive organs, which need spaciousness in the abdominal cavity to function optimally. Imagine someone squeezing you very tightly and demanding that you do your best in a relaxed and efficient way. That could be very challenging, to say the least!

All of the armors in our bodies, and specifically the abdominal one, keep us from receiving and acting on intuition, our voice of guidance. It is essential that we "let our guards down" with ourselves so we can ground in a sense of self, listen for our inner guidance, and act accordingly. As author and teacher Caroline Myss writes, "The ability to glean intuitive guidance from one's own spirit rests on a strong sense of self and on respect for that self."[4]

In the Womb-Dantian, you can access a point of light that can grow into a sun, reaching its zenith in your heart. The degree of radiance and subsequent amplitude of this sun rest upon how you feel about yourself. The more you regard yourself—including your body—with love, kindness, and respect, the warmer, more radiantly, and expansively the sun will shine within you and out into the world, and the more glorious your dance will become. This is exactly why, when you don't feel good about yourself, the world outside appears dim and gloomy. The brightness you perceive outside always mirrors the brightness you cultivate inside. Rumi alludes to this truth when he says, "Life is the sound of your inner voice."[5] What you experience in life are your own thoughts and feelings echoed back to you. They either magnify the radiance of the sun in your center or darken it.

A healthy sense of self goes hand in hand with the development of the sun in your center. It allows you to set appropriate boundaries and take full responsibility for your life, enabling the rays of your inner sun to shine even in the places where you once felt victimized so you can live the mantra "I AM the only authority in my world." The "I AM" presence refers to the divine spark or consciousness that exists within every individual and all that exists. It is your connection to the infinite, eternal source of life, often described as the higher self, divine self, or source within. Rooted in many spiritual traditions, the "I AM" is recognized as the true essence of a person, transcending the ego and limited mind.

Cultivating this presence begins with accepting yourself exactly as you are, while also acknowledging the areas you struggle to accept and dedicating yourself to healing them so that self-acceptance can blossom into appreciation and even love. This is not an overnight process. Remember to proceed with kindness and adab (soul courtesy) toward yourself, even when you uncover your most "dreadful" shadows.

How you feel about yourself and the respect you hold for yourself directly influence the quality of your life, including your success in business, relationships, and healing. As Caroline Myss affirms:

> Self-understanding and acceptance, the bond we form with ourselves, is in many ways the most crucial spiritual challenge we face. In truth, if we do not like ourselves, we will be incapable of making healthy decisions. . . . People who have a low sense of self-esteem attract relationships and occupational situations that reflect and reinforce this weakness.[6]

In this light, the relationships and circumstances you attract are not punishments, but teachers—mirrors that reveal what needs healing in you so that self-esteem can deepen. To strengthen this foundation, cultivate practices that build power in the Womb-Dantian: take responsibility, live with discipline, keep your promises, complete what you begin, refuse excuses, and refrain from blaming others for how you feel. Others may wrong you, but how you respond to their actions is entirely within your power.

Discipline, tempered with compassion, is essential. The practice that follows will help you cultivate the strength of your Womb-Dantian and center yourself in genuine self-esteem.

THE SUN IN YOUR CENTER
with video component

This practice can be done daily or three times per week as you begin your Dance of Oneness training. You can do it after the Basic Meditation practice (chapter 4) or on its own.

Time required: 10–30 minutes

> Stand with bare feet, either indoors or outside on grass, in a quiet, secluded area. Place your feet shoulder-width apart, parallel to each other. Soften your knees and release your tailbone downward toward the Earth without tucking your spine forward. Let your low back remain in a neutral position. Allow yourself to feel gratitude and appreciation for your surroundings.

> Make loose fists and become aware of where your ring and middle fingers touch your palm. The area on your palm where

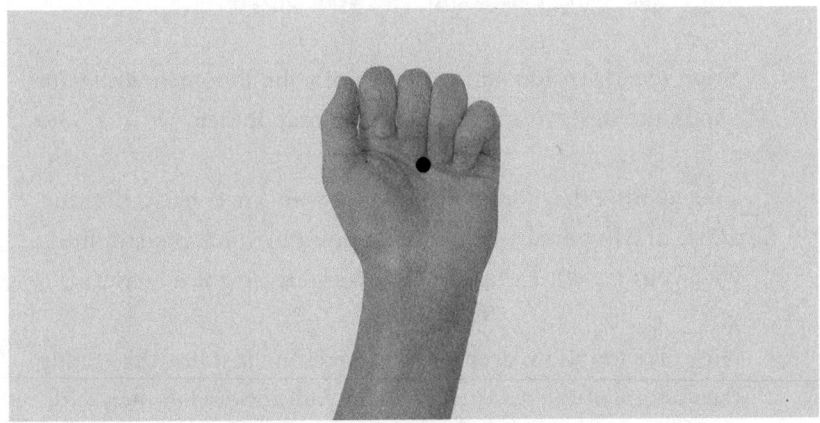

FIGURE 6. Lao Gong meridian point in the center of the palm

the tips of your middle and ring fingers naturally touch is where the meridian point known as Lao Gong (Palace of Toil) is located (see Figure 6). Used for healing work and Qigong, stimulating this point has many benefits, including easing anxiety and building internal power. Use the thumb of your right hand to stimulate this point in your left palm by making small circles for about one minute. Repeat on the other hand.

Look at the diagram of the inverted cone showing the Womb-Dantian (see Figure 5).

Place your palms on your lower abdomen, creating a downward facing triangle, with the tips of your thumbs meeting on your navel. Sense the Lao Gong points in your palms. Close your eyes and come in touch with the inverted cone on your lower belly.

Take a deep breath. As you inhale through your nose, expand your belly outward.

Exhale through your nose, softening your belly gently inward, releasing your weight further down. Awaken the soles of your feet to the living Earth, and relax your hips.

Sense the expansion and softening of your abdomen with your hands and observe any tension in your abdomen.

Take another deep breath, and sense your lower back. Become aware of Mingmen (the meridian point in your spine, in line with your navel). Exhale and release your weight downward.

Now take ten more deep breaths, each one just like this, filling the volume of the inverted cone on your lower abdomen with your breath and awareness. Each time, allow your belly to soften more, sensing this softening in your hands.

Now, ask yourself: How do I feel in this part of my body? Can I be here with ease?

Start to feel as though you are holding yourself like a baby. If you cannot nurture and protect yourself, and feel secure within, you will not find true nurture and protection anywhere in the outside world.

Soften your belly so it feels as if your fingers can enter into your belly. You are beginning to soften your abdominal armor. Trust yourself. (Even if you feel like the external layer of your abdomen is "flabby," there is most likely a hardness in the deeper layers).

The lower tip of the triangle, where your index fingers are touching and moving in, extends into your Womb-Dantian. Located deep inside in the center of the inverted cone, your Womb-Dantian is accessed through relaxing the outer layer of your abdomen and awareness in your lower back (the area of Mingmen).

Feel into your Womb-Dantian for a couple minutes. See if you can envision a point of light here. This is how you yourself began in the womb of your mother.

Inhale and feel the point of light grow bigger, into a ball of light that encompasses your whole Womb-Dantian. Exhale, staying in touch with this ball of light, and release your tailbone downward.

Take two more breaths, feeling the ball of light in your Womb-Dantian.

Inhale and feel the ball of light expand into rays that fill your whole lower abdomen.

Exhale, focusing the rays back into the ball of light in your Womb-Dantian, and sense your tailbone releasing downward.

Repeat the same pattern of inhaling, allowing the light to expand in your body gradually, and exhaling, as you focus the rays back into the ball of light in your Womb-Dantian. Visualize the ball of light in your Womb-Dantian as the center of the sun, with its rays emanating into your entire body.

Start slowly rocking forward and backward as you take deep breaths. Inhale as you rock forward, bringing your weight over the balls of your feet. And as you exhale, return to neutral, shifting your weight evenly onto the soles of your feet.

Monitor your abdomen with your hands so it doesn't begin to tighten. Stay relaxed and supple. Repeat the rocking motion five times.

On your sixth time rocking forward, slowly take your hands off your abdomen, keeping them about three inches in front of your belly. In your hands, feel the warmth and the emanation of the sun from your Womb-Dantian.

Rock backward and slowly bring your hands back onto your belly.

Sensing the center of your sun and its rays extending into your whole body, slowly take your hands off your belly and keep them about three inches in front of your abdomen. Turn your palms to face each other, but keep them approximately three inches apart. Sense the Lao Gong points in your palms and a connection between the two points (see Figure 7). If you need a reminder of the points' location, make a loose fist and focus on the area in your palms between where the tips of your ring and middle fingers touch.

With your next inhalation, as you expand the rays of the sun in your center, gently extend your palms outward toward the sides of your abdomen—as if your arms were naturally extending as a result of your abdomen's expansion.

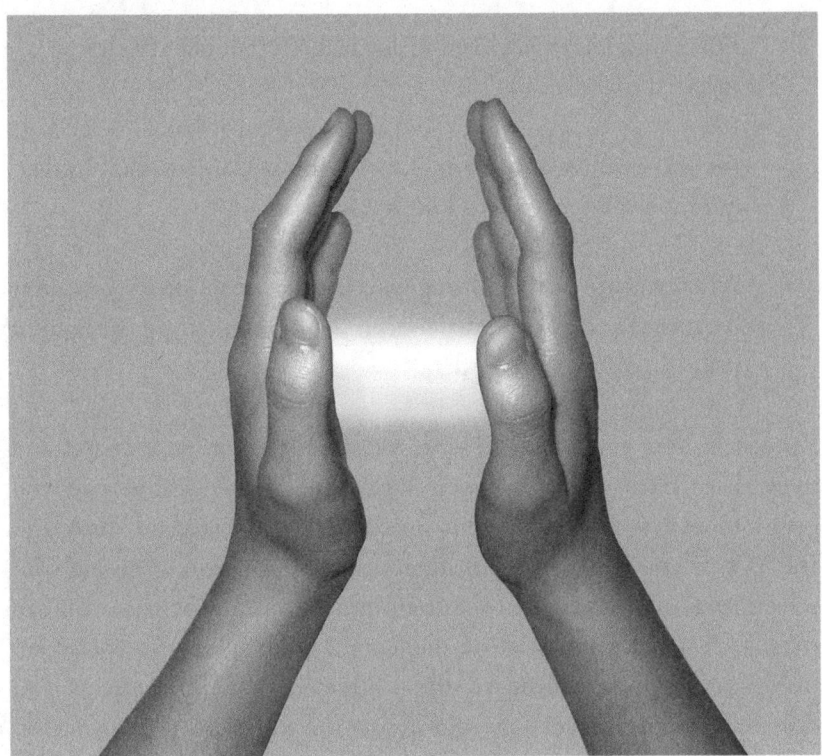

FIGURE 7. The energy between the two Lao Gong points in your palm

Exhale and return your palms back to about three inches apart. Focus your energy back into the center of your sun. Repeat this five times.

Next, inhale and lift your arms to the level of your shoulders, keeping the points in your palms connected. Feel the rays of the sun in your center extend into your whole abdomen, heart center, shoulders, arms, and hands.

Exhale and bring your palms to the original position of about three inches apart. Focus your energy back into the center of your sun. Repeat this five times.

Bring your hands back onto your belly in the shape of the inverted triangle.

Sense the center of the sun in your Womb-Dantian. Rest in this luminous presence for as long as you wish.

When you are ready to bring your practice to a close, take a deep breath in, and as you exhale, open your eyes—letting the light of your inner sun shine forth.

Reflect on how you extended your movements from your center and drew them back to your center. When you move in this way, you begin to experience movement as energizing instead of depleting. This is how you begin to cultivate your center. Instead of giving your power away or letting it leak out from a lack of awareness, you can trace a clear path of initiating movement from the source of power inside you and returning to the source. This practice helps you develop "staying power" in your center so you can begin to feel at home within yourself.

∞

PRACTICE

INNER SMILE

with audio component

This practice supports you in developing ease in your body and a deeper love for yourself. You can do it after the Sun in Your Center practice or on its own.

Time required: 5–15 minutes

Bring your hands together in the shape of the inverted triangle on your belly. Close your eyes.

Become aware of the center of the sun in your Womb-Dantian.

As you breathe through your nose, see if you can come in touch with a smile in the center of the sun.

Once you can feel this smile, begin to radiate it into your sexual organs, bladder, genitals, hips, legs, knees, feet, and in the Earth through your body. Feel how smiling in these parts of your body brings ease.

Now, smile in your intestines, stomach, liver, gallbladder, and kidneys, giving gratitude to your organs for their meticulous work.

Now, smile up your spine to the nape of your neck and the back of your head.

Smile in your heart, your lungs, and into your shoulders, arms, and hands.

Smile in your neck, face, eyes, and ears.

Let your lips form into a broad smile. Feel the smile filling your whole body, softly expressed through your lips. Let yourself feel gratitude for your miraculous body and glorious being.

Feel your beauty from the inside.

Say, "I love you" to yourself (and take note of any discomfort or difficulty that arises as you say these words).

Say, "I am as the Beloved has created me" to yourself.

Observe how you feel. Do you feel empowered and elated, like nothing in the outside world could contain or limit your power?

When you're ready, bring the practice to a close by opening your eyes and allowing your inner smile to emanate from your eyes.

Observe any changes in your sight. Do your surroundings appear clearer, the colors more vivid? As Rumi asks,

Why is the rose laughing?
It is because she is holding her flowerness in her hands
and smelling it abundantly,
filling her senses with her own perfume.[7]

What is your unique "ness"—the special quality that only you bring into the world? Add "ness" to the end of your name, and create spontaneous dance moves as you say or sing your name with this suffix.

Let your body guide you into stillness when the time is right.

Remember to smile when you are in a stressful situation and observe how it can relax you, disarm others, and help you deal with the situation more effectively.

Another effective soothing gesture to use in challenging, stressful times is to put one hand or both hands on your heart, with the awareness of the Lao Gong points in your palms, as a way of embracing, nurturing, and filling yourself with love.

∞

THE SMILE

At the end of my sessions, people often ask me, "How can I remember all the things you've taught us? How am I going to remember, especially in those moments when it's difficult?" "Smile," is my response, "and let the smile relax you into feeling your beauty and the radiance that lives in you."

In her book *Talking with Angels*, Gitta Mallasz writes, "The smile is the prayer of every cell . . . the inner smile is the first condition for becoming HUMAN."[8] It is very important to cultivate this inner smile as we just did in our practice smiling through your very organs, muscles, and sinews, bathing yourself in ease, relaxation, peace, and acceptance—while honoring, and loving yourself exactly as you are. "Have you ever noticed where you actually are when you are unable to smile? You are in the mud, up to your neck in the mire, or even to the crown of your head."[9] It is in these moments that we need to smile from our depths and see how it shifts everything.

Remember that your relationship with yourself forms the basis of all your relationships and how you navigate life.

Having explored the foundational energies of the first six rays of Dance of Oneness—in correspondence with the first three chakras—we have laid the groundwork for embodiment. From cultivating presence in the body to grounding in the Earth, from recognizing ourselves as channels of energy to embracing our sexuality as a sacred life force, and, finally, centering and moving from a place of self-love and inner alignment, these principles form the essence of our dance.

Next, we will turn to the great streams of wisdom that have nourished the spirit of Dance of Oneness: flamenco, Tai Chi, and the Gurdjieff Work. Each tradition carries a profound understanding of energy, presence, and transformation, expressed in its own unique language of movement. Together, they offer pathways for embodying the first six rays and for deepening our journey into embodied awakening.

9

FIRE OF FLAMENCO

Alchemize the Shadow
and Heal from Trauma

Integration of Rays 1–6

We begin with flamenco—a dance form that embodies the first six rays we have explored, with a special emphasis on the last: "loving who you are." Flamenco is a sacred fire, a powerful current of movement that awakens sovereignty and self-authority. Rooted in the Earth, it engages the three Chakras of Matter—the Root, Sacral, and Solar Plexus—igniting sexual energy as a source of strength and shaping a vibrant sense of self.

Flamenco was the first dance modality in which I trained. From the very first time I saw it, I knew instantly—this was my dance! I had found a form I longed to devote myself to with all my being, and at the same time, I felt as if I had been dancing it all my life.

Part of why it possessed me at first sight was that it is an expression of the Roma, a people who are constantly moving, going from one place and culture to another. Flamenco is a hybrid form, a great meeting of the East and the West, emerging from a people migrating from India through the Middle East, Eastern Europe, and North Africa to finally settle in Spain. It is the expression of outsiders who had to become self-reliant and sovereign in an unknown environment. When I found it, I had recently left Iran for the United States. I was like a Roma woman in search of her identity, and flamenco became my mirror—reflecting back my inner state, with all the anger, frustration, and grief simmering within me, ready to erupt, longing to find expression and give voice to my story.

Flamenco expressed what I longed to learn, both as a dance and as a way of life, which was to cultivate a sensual yet strong, noble, and dignified presence as a woman. It was like I was breathing in a new kind of air when I saw how unashamed the flamenco dancer is of her own power and how authentic and unapologetic she is. She doesn't have to impress anyone or even smile unless that is *truly* how she feels.

At the time, I was filled with rage and sorrow. It was no accident that the first dance to speak to my heart—the one that helped me begin to bear the agony of my condition and find release from the paralysis and silencing my traumas had inflicted—was the ferocious flamenco. Through it, I could transform my pain, anger, and deep grief into art. It was inevitable that I would choose the most vehement, fierce, and naked form to transmute the energies of my suffering into offering, ecstasy, and praise. I experienced flamenco as both a howl for freedom and a furnace I could plunge myself into for purification.

Later, at age twenty, when I was an undergraduate at the University of California, Irvine (UCI), destiny brought me face-to-face with my beloved flamenco teacher, Antonia Rojas Kabakov—my second dance teacher after the Divine.

My passion for flamenco helped me excel quickly. Barely into my second year of training, Antonia invited me to join the UCI Spanish Dance Ensemble, and I became a lead dancer. When a local guitarist sought a dancer for a gig at a Spanish restaurant, Antonia chose me. Though nervous about performing solo, she reminded me that flamenco is fundamentally a solo dance and urged me to seize the opportunity.

I began my first professional gig. The setup was far from glamorous—a cramped office served as my dressing room, and I navigated a hot, greasy kitchen before stepping on stage. My nerves were high, and the guitarist's rhythm faltered, but the spirit of flamenco carried me. The audience applauded wildly, though the uninspiring music and out-of-tune playing soon became hard to ignore. Too shy to confront the guitarist, I continued performing, but each gig left me more anxious. By the third performance, the smelly kitchen and lewd bar patrons made me feel out of place. As I danced, I heard a voice say, "This is not my place. I don't want any part of this." It was the spirit of dance herself.

The restaurant gig ended abruptly. Despite offers of more money, I quit, knowing my allegiance was to dance. Since then, I've refused performances where the music or environment doesn't honor the spirit of dance.

Flamenco empowered me to be real about my needs. It requires authenticity, discipline, and full alignment with the music. After leaving the restaurant gig, I returned to the ensemble with renewed dedication. The more I learned and performed, the more elated, confident, powerful, and sensually magnetic I became as a performer and a woman.

DARKNESS IS MY CANDLE

Flamenco is an initiation into the dark aspects of the Divine Feminine that urge us to embrace our inner depths, face our fears, and transform. It is a journey into the agony and ecstasy of a being who incarnates and lives the chaos and glory of being alive with wild nobility. She is passionate, ferocious and wild, yet mysterious, out of reach, and austere. As the primal undercurrent of all that is, the dark aspects of the Divine Feminine came into my world to ignite me with the raw power and volcanic energy that rises from the Earth's molten core, forging rubies from the depths of the soil.

Through flamenco, the Divine Feminine guided me to set my darkness on fire, to dance it, and to be enlivened by it—to move through the forbidden emotions of shame, anger, and resentment rather than deny or suppress them, letting them burn me in their dark fire. I was set ablaze, becoming an alchemical vessel where dark and light could come together.

Flamenco teaches us to withstand life's challenges with wild nobility—to hold both the joy and the pain as inseparable dance partners, to let wild grace inspire and carry us, remain untamed, never overcome! Love, too, is both joy and pain.

FIRST INITIATION: TRANSMUTE SHADOW CONTENT INTO ART

Flamenco burned me, but it also gave me immeasurable initiations over time—gifts I offer you as five fundamental teachings of embodiment that can be applied to both dance and life. These initiations lie at the core of Dance of Oneness. The first initiation is about the importance of transmuting your shadow into art, transforming it into something life-affirming through creativity. In flamenco, pain, grief, suffering, anger, and fear are alchemized into dance and music. The invitation is not to cower in fear or tremble before calamity, but to dance it, to give it voice, and to let it become your strength. Flamenco empowers us to *dance* our rage and sorrow, and shows us how important it is to not repress them. Destructive energies need not frighten us; they can be harnessed for fierce creation. This is the path to activating a body of light. Dancing the darkness helped me break through to the light of love, and it can do the same for you.

All of our experiences and feelings are material for our creativity and growth. And it is specifically the dark places that we need to reach into within ourselves in order to find the creative life and nourish it. Darkness guides us to find our inner gifts. As Clarissa Pinkola Estés writes, "The dark is not a horrible place but a place of gifts and treasure."[1]

This is the way in which we refuse to allow the outside world to overpower, tame, or break us. Instead of letting pain and grief engulf us or letting anger, exhaustion, and fear freeze us, we keep moving. We dance the darkness. We dance to free ourselves from oppression. Clarissa shares this about flamenco:

> It is a dance that came out of not being pristine, came out of
> not being free, and as a result the soul was made free, the soul
> burst free, and not only for the people who danced the dance
> and who made the music, but in the people who were the
> listeners and the people who were the watchers of it.[2]

Flamenco illustrates a triumphant journey through pain and suffering. The triumph comes from fully living and expressing that pain until, at last, you break free. When you use adversity as an opening to creativity, you have triumphed. The full cycle of this journey must be lived and expressed in the dance, or there is no catharsis, no deliverance. Without pain and suffering, triumph is meaningless. Flamenco is the form through which we can express anger, frustration, and fear—and in the end, arrive at joy. Soleares, or Deep Song, begins at the height of grief and ends with Bulerías, which comes from the Spanish word "burlar" (to mock) and "bullería" (racket, shouting, din). This is the liberation that comes from living and owning the dark, transforming you into the "rend"—the Sufi "trickster"—master of paradox. For the Sufis, a rend is one who faces their inner darkness, acknowledging and integrating the shadow without judgment. Unbound and free from societal expectations or the need to appear "good" or virtuous, the rend challenge rigid structures by transcending dualities and embracing life's paradoxes.

In the same way, flamenco shows us that liberation from the dark comes only by entering it—by finding its noble essence, and discovering its pure rawness. Through fully expressing the darkness and transmuting it into fierce beauty and art, we become embodied and exhilarated with the joy of life, a joy vast enough to embrace even the most extreme forms of suffering. For example, by beginning with a posture that represents total restriction, we can slowly, painfully, and with effort and grace begin to open and eventually arrive at a state of thriving, passionately pulsating with aliveness.

So, in a sense, flamenco teaches us the fierce psychological alchemy that is required for the embodiment process. It is not a matter of denying or suppressing difficult emotions, as happens in patriarchal mystical systems. Rather, it calls us to face them, uncover their source, and tap into their vital energy. This brings a sense of wholeness capable of embracing everything—saying yes to life, and knowing again and again the price of that yes. It is a path of nobility and integrity, of accepting life as the atrocious, beautiful, violating, and rebirthing experience that it always is.

And you are not concerned about not appearing *pretty* because you couldn't care less about *pretty*. Pretty is too small and confining. In flamenco, you express the difficult emotions within the form of a glorious lion-wolf-bull-hawk-crow being—a sculpture of rules. Flamenco offers a geometry that arises from an archaic mystery: inner discipline and a sacredly structured container allow you to bear anything and transmute whatever atrocity you have endured—or may face in the future—into deeper courage, greater dignity, and a more ferocious embrace of life. This is why it is essential to have a dedicated practice like Dance of Oneness, a way of cultivating your body and being as a sacred container that can withstand life's challenges.

Sometimes the audience will hurl the worst obscenities at flamenco performers—as compliments. It's wild, a fusion of obscenity and transcendence, akin to what the Sufis call "kharabat" (the tavern of ruin): finding the holy in the dung. It is a fierce marriage of opposites.

Nobility is embedded in the very structure of flamenco, in its sacred geometry, born of discipline. This is a living, fiery geometry—so even in obscenity, there is grace, because it is archetypal. And when anger erupts in flamenco, it is not merely personal; it is the anger of confronting injustice and deception.

SECOND INITIATION: KEEPER OF THE FLAME

Flamenco is a dance of fire. To dance this form, you need to come in touch with your essential spark, which can grow into a flame through discipline and grace. Flamenco is about tending to this flame and keeping it alive, sometimes guarding it under your cape so the wind doesn't put it out, especially when it is young. The second initiation Flamenco offers is the recognition that, as keepers of the flame, we must learn to tend it skillfully—fanning the fire when needed and tempering its intensity with wisdom. Flamenco teaches us to dance the fine line between too much fire, which can burn us and others, and too little fire, which leaves everyone frozen, lifeless, and disengaged.

What I learned from flamenco became the backbone of my dance—the actual chalice. In the beginning, I danced and practiced for six to seven hours every day. I was dedicated to mastering the lines, the precision, the geometric shapes, the very architecture of Flamenco. This was not the time to indulge in emotions. It was a meticulous crafting of form, so that when I poured my anger, agony, and sorrow into these geometric shapes, I was pouring them into an alchemical crucible. In flamenco, you don't express your shadow at random; it must gestate to become profound and meaningful, like a piece by Ludwig van Beethoven. There is a science at work here—the science of disciplined precision in the alchemical process of transmutation.

What flamenco gives us is a total and absolute sense of how rigor, precision, and intense commitment to the purity of the form are the requirements on the path of dance. Many modalities today claim to be sacred dance, yet they do not begin with a true focus on the language and technique of dance. When I speak of the "language of dance," I am not talking about expressing whatever is our whim or fancy. Self-expression is vital, but it is most powerful when it moves within form—within discipline and structure. Form is as important as the content expressed. In flamenco, there is a marriage of opposites: uncompromising rigor, with a foundation that demands everything of you, joined with the unleashing of the wildest possible imagination.

Anyone, not just a dancer, can benefit from this teaching. The principle of tending to the flame—nurturing our inner spark with discipline and care—applies to all aspects of life. Whether in art, work, relationships, or personal growth, the balance between rigor and passion is essential. Too much intensity can lead to burnout, while too little can leave us uninspired and disengaged. By committing to a practice with devotion and precision, we create a container strong enough to hold our deepest emotions and transmute them into something meaningful. This is the alchemy of mastery, available to anyone willing to tend their inner fire.

THIRD INITIATION: HONOR YOUR SEXUALITY

The third initiation invites you to own and honor your sexuality. This is the seat of your life force. You can be sensual and luscious to the degree you are comfortable with, without over-eroticizing or selling yourself to please anyone. As the keeper of the flame, you are the ruler of your own realm. This principle is essential in empowering you to feel simultaneously sensual and strong without shame or judgment.

In flamenco, a woman is free to be herself exactly as she wishes, on her own terms. She is celebrated for her strength, dignity, passion, wildness, audacity, courage, and vulnerability. The more real and sovereign she is, the more she is cherished.

FOURTH INITIATION: NEVER BE OVERPOWERED!

The fourth initiation of flamenco is the refusal to let anything in the outside world overpower, break, or tame you. To dance flamenco is to be wild yet noble, dignified, and sovereign. Echoing the second initiation—the need to balance too much and too little fire—this path is cultivated through confidence, courage, and self-reliance.

The invitation is to hold your self-worth in your gaze and never diminish yourself in the company of others. Instead, stay rooted in your wild nobility, drawing inspiration from flamenco's totem animals: hawk, crow, bull, wolf, and lion. Many of us are lions who mistake ourselves for sheep; flamenco awakens the solar energy within us—the true lion.

Flamenco is a training in the manner of the great Iranian mystic Shams-e Tabrizi, Rumi's teacher and beloved companion. Shams (whose name means "the Sun" in Arabic) was a solar being, initiating seekers into their true self through a fierce fire—precisely the fire needed for alchemy. Described as a black lion, he embodied nobility, ferocity, and a discerning sovereignty. Approaching flamenco in the spirit of Shams, we too are initiated into courage and nobility.

It is also important to remember flamenco's profound Middle Eastern influence. Like Sufi whirling, it shatters the chains of bondage we impose on ourselves. The path of flamenco is akin to that of the ghalandar (wandering darvish)—free, uninhibited, and irrepressible, like Shams himself. Rumi describes the ghalandar-like state in this way:

> I've come again, I've come again,
> I've come from the Beloved.
> Look at me, gaze deeply into me,

I've come to console you.
I've come in joy, I've come in joy,
I've come free from all attachments.[3]

In the first verse, Rumi uses the Persian word "baaz" (again). "Baaz" has several other meanings as well. One meaning is "hawk," another is "open," and yet another is "play." Rumi uses all four meanings. So, in the first verse, he is saying, "I've come again," "I've come as a hawk," "I've come free," and "I've come playfully" all at once. In another poem, he says,

You are like a hawk
whose feet are tethered,
weighed down by the body;
it's with your own hands
that you must untie the knots.[4]

Flamenco reminds us that we are hawks who are meant to be free. It shows us how to untie the knots that weigh us down, and it invites us to be playful. When I teach flamenco, I guide people to feel and hold their own power, to awaken a sense of wild nobility in themselves. I always remind them, "You are neither greater nor lesser than anyone else." Power is a tricky domain that one must tread with responsibility and awareness. True power is sovereignty within yourself—power that inspires others to awaken to their own. It arises in proportion to how aligned we are with the Beloved and how freely we allow the life force to move through us.

A student once told me, "You are one of the few women I have met who is not only *not* threatened by another woman's beauty and greatness, but actually celebrates it." Flamenco taught me this. If you and I are dancing together and I shrink back because I think you are more beautiful than I am, I cannot show up fully in my own dance. Flamenco is generous in that it grants entry to anyone lit up by passion, but it is also exacting. To dance flamenco, you must arrive poised, with everything you've got—physically beautiful or not. There is no room for holding back. If you defer to comparison—*so and so is more beautiful than me, or they're a better dancer than me*—you cannot do your thing. You're lost. You'll be told, "Next please. Let the one who *knows* her own worth take the stage."

This lesson extends far beyond flamenco; it's a call for us all to step into our power. Whether in art, work, relationships, or daily living, knowing your true worth and self-assurance are what empower you to show up fully and serve the greater good.

Flamenco is where we confront our self-sabotaging fears and shyness, those born not of true humility but of neurosis. As Rumi says: "If you're a lover of love, take a dagger to the throat of your shyness and forced modesty."[5]

There is architecture at play here—a structure that cultivates discernment. Flamenco's movements are defined and clearly articulated, carving precise delineations in space. Many of the arm movements and positions signify breaking chains and releasing oneself from bondage. In this way, the dance trains us to dissolve confining boundaries and create new ones. These movements shape our identity and instill responsibility and sovereignty—reminding us that we are free, not victims.

FIFTH INITIATION: FIND DUENDE

Flamenco is both mythic and universal, yet unique to the individual. Once you pass through the initial stages of training, you are encouraged to cultivate and express your uniqueness. This uniqueness is woven from the threads and themes of your life, and from the audacity, courage, creativity, stamina, and discipline you bring to transforming them into art.

This brings us to the fifth initiation flamenco offers: the importance of duende (spirit). If there is any clue to the essence of flamenco, it lies in this mystery. Duende is both the mother and the child of the previous four initiations. When we dare to enter the dark to recover our inner flame, and when we refuse to be tamed or overpowered, duende awakens in us and dances through us. It magnifies our spark, keeps us wild yet noble, and guides us through the shadows to uncover the hidden gold within.

There's an essay on duende by Spanish writer Federico García Lorca, in which he writes, "Seeking the duende, there is neither map nor discipline. We only know it burns the blood like powdered glass . . . baptizing all who gaze at it with dark water."[6]

It takes everything you have to become a great flamenco artist. To be a flamenco dancer requires a disciplined body, a fierce and passionate soul, and a heart willing to expose its deepest heartbreak and greatest vulnerability. It calls for someone who can hold turmoil within a lucid, peaceful structure through an almost impossibly demanding discipline. You must balance total audacity with total discipline. This is an all-or-nothing endeavor: you either give yourself completely, or forget it. You can't go halfway. You practice tirelessly to chisel and shape your instrument so you're ready, so you're available for grace. Pain is what makes you available. Then you step aside, and duende takes over. The goal is *to be danced*. In order to be danced, you have to have created the dancer who is disciplined enough and softened enough in a grueling marriage of opposites.

"Being danced" means allowing the music, the rhythm, or a greater force to move through you—guiding your body in a way that feels organic and unforced, as if you are being moved rather than moving yourself. From a spiritual perspective, something you can apply not just to dance but to your life, it means to release resistance, to trust in the process, and to become a vessel for something beyond yourself.

In flamenco, discipline and form provide the container for the enormous power that arrives when you marry fidelity to the craft with fearless abandon to the moment and the emotion that is being born in you. What emerges is a ferocious beauty—wild, noble, uncompromising, disruptive, bold, fierce, engaged, present, available, and alert. To watch true flamenco is to see spirit incarnate itself in matter, stripped of illusion and prettifying masks. You are witnessing life naked, raw, and untamed.

Flamenco's totem animals are the lion, wolf, bull, hawk, and crow. I include the crow because flamenco is not about conventional beauty. It carries a raw awkwardness and a glimmering, mysterious quality, like the crow itself. Flamenco is ragged and intense, as imperfect as it is perfect. If you appear too perfect, polished and flawless, you are not dancing flamenco— you are trying too hard. Lions, wolves, bulls, and hawks embody natural perfection; they cannot help but be beautiful. But we also drive ourselves into ugly corners and razor-sharp places, and flamenco embraces this. It hungers for it, declaring: "I'm not afraid of the ugly, bring on the ugly. I'm not afraid of suffering. I can take it as long as I can dance it."

This teaches us that true power and beauty are born in the balance between discipline and raw, unfiltered expression. Flamenco reminds us that life is not about polished perfection but about meeting intensity, imperfection, and even struggle with courage and presence. Like flamenco, we come alive when we stop fearing the rough edges of living and instead dance with them—boldly, fiercely, and fully alive.

BEWARE ALL YE WHO ENTER!

As much as flamenco helps us cultivate a strong sense of self and sovereignty, some say it can also lead to an inflated ego. At the time, I lacked the psychic and spiritual maturity to hold the level of energy moving through me, and I set out to cultivate it in myself only after the fact. When I danced flamenco, I became powerful and magnetic—but without grounding or awareness. Inevitably, I burned. Drama erupted in almost every area of my life. As I said earlier, flamenco is a dance of fire: if you do not know how to tend the flame, it will consume you. Yet it is precisely through burning that you learn to tend it. As Rumi says, "It is by entering into the heart of fire that you become a butterfly."[7]

I seemed to have no other choice but to enter right into the heart of the fire. At the height of my dancing prowess, conflicts with Antonia, my teacher and company director, reached an unbearable peak. We were preparing our biggest staging to date. As prima soloist, I was featured in most of the dances, and for the first time I had been asked to choreograph my own solo. But just a week before opening night, tensions forced me to withdraw from the show. It devastated the company—most of all, me. To abandon a production at that stage is the greatest taboo in my field, and I had unfortunately committed it.

Soon after, through my own recklessness, I also lost the man I considered the love of my life, a partner of two years I had expected to marry. At barely twenty-four, my life unraveled. The fire of flamenco consumed me, and I could no longer dance it. The power was too intense and held so much sexual magnetism. Men and women alike gravitated to me. I had power over them, but I had no idea how to carry it. It was frightening, and the other dancers resented me. "Why does *she* get all the main parts?" they asked. Jealousy and drama surrounded me, mirroring the very drama inherent in flamenco itself.

I no longer understood where all the power in me was coming from or what it was for. I started to question it. Was it my ego? I had uncovered the shadow of flamenco in myself as pride, self-absorption, and destructive vanity. I could no longer hold my head high and declare, "Yes, I can take it." I was shattered, unsure who I was anymore. I withdrew from flamenco altogether and stopped performing.

Looking back, I see I was being shown what a life of fame without grounding in divine service looks like. As dazzling and glamorous as it seemed, it was not for me. I could not be a diva blissed out on my own greatness. I was meant to be both empress *and* servant. I had lost my way and needed to find my way back to the Beloved again.

Flamenco taught me how to confront myself. With great agony and remorse, I pleaded: "Is this who I really am?" When grace revealed that this was only one of my faces, I softened and sighed, "Thank Goddess, can I now be shown another face please?!"

PRACTICE

LOOKING AT YOURSELF IN A MIRROR
with audio component

This practice awakens two of flamenco's hidden gifts. The first is the embrace of yourself as you are—inhabiting your body with love, dignity, and presence. The second is the power of a steady gaze, learning to rest your eyes and attention upon one point without wavering. Return to this practice once a month for six months. You may weave it in after The Sun in Your Center practice (chapter 8), or let it stand on its own. After each practice, take time to reflect on your experience and journal.

Time required: 10–20 minutes each time over three days

Sit or stand naked in front of a mirror. Begin by gazing into your own eyes for at least three minutes, simply noticing how you feel. Allow any judgments, criticisms, or complaints to arise and let them be voiced. Observe them without trying to change them.

Expand your gaze to take in your whole face. Notice your judgments, your likes and dislikes. Ask yourself if you can accept your face as it is. If you find that you cannot, gently observe what you would like to be different. Ask where this desire comes from—perhaps from something someone once said, something you absorbed from your culture, or from your feelings about aging. Is it something superficial, like a blemish or wrinkles, or is it deeper and not easily remedied? Give yourself space to discover why acceptance feels hard in this place.

Roll your shoulders back and down a few times, then loosen your neck and torso by swaying side to side. Shake out your arms and hands, then your legs and feet.

Move for as long as you need, and come into stillness when your body naturally settles. Take three deep Love Breaths.

Close your eyes and awaken the soles of your feet to the pulse of the living Earth. Place your hands in the inverted triangle position on your lower abdomen, sensing the Lao Gong points in your palms. Focus your breathing into your Womb-Dantian. Do the Inner Smile practice (chapter 8).

When you are ready, open your eyes, smiling directly into your own eyes. Say to yourself, "I love you."

Then say, "I am as the Beloved has created me."

Blow yourself a kiss.

When you are ready, take a few minutes to write down the feelings and insights that arose.

On the following day, repeat this practice, this time focusing on your upper body and torso. On the next day, return again, focusing on the lower part of your body, below the waist. Continue until you have made peace with your entire body.

When you revisit this practice later, you may choose to do a whole-body scan at once. Keep your notes together so you can witness how your relationship with yourself and your body grows and evolves over time.

∞

The sixth ray of Dance of Oneness invites you into a loving, sovereign relationship with yourself and your body—a strength that rises from within. Yet sovereignty on its own is not the whole story. Just as fire's intensity is tempered by water's coolness, self-authority finds its true power when joined with humility. In the next chapter, we enter this dance of opposites—sovereignty and humility, fire and water—and discover how their union opens the way to deeper harmony.

10

TAI CHI

The Way of Water

Integration of Rays 1–6

Flamenco puro, which I danced, is an all-or-nothing endeavor. There is no middle ground. It totally empowered me and totally destroyed me. It was great heartbreak that propelled me beyond it. I floated around in confusion and despair until one day, quite unexpectedly, I ran into a group of people in a park doing very slow movements in unison. I watched their entire routine in utter amazement. When I danced alone, I loved moving like them—in a slow, drawn-out tempo.

This was my first encounter with Tai Chi, and my reaction was exactly the same as when I first saw flamenco. Here was a modality I wanted to study with all my being, yet I felt I had always moved in this way. Though my reactions to Tai Chi may have resembled those I had to flamenco, the modality and lifestyle I was entering were worlds apart.

Like flamenco, Tai Chi also embodies the first six rays of Dance of Oneness. It engages all three Chakras of Matter—the Root, Sacral, and Solar Plexus Chakras—as it is a grounded form of movement that harmonizes the dual energies of yin and yang and helps us cultivate the Womb-Dantian as our powerhouse.

In Tai Chi, I found the middle ground I had been missing from the all-or-nothing world of flamenco. I went from having the proud face of the lioness—the wild, devouring feline who held her power and self-worth in her gaze and stomped with determination and will—to completely melting my identity into the greater mystery.

A lioness needs balance and emptiness so as not to be consumed by her imperial power. The keeper of the flame is not the flame itself. After the initiation into the molten power of the dark feminine and the ferocious solar masculine, I needed soothing. Faced with the intensity of fire, you either learn to find balance or you burn out. I was burned, charred, and in need of water's cooling balm. I longed to be submerged in unknowing because flamenco really *knows*. All the cries of passion and eros, the howl of the primordial and unbounded human, needed to dissolve into the formless—the unknowing silence. I was too full; I needed to become empty and humble.

REEEELAXXXX

After studying with a couple of teachers, I eventually found Dr. Wong, a master of Tai Chi and Qigong. Watching him do Tai Chi for the very first time brought tears to my eyes—it was one of the most beautiful dances I had ever seen. He spoke very little English and knew only a few key words. The one he emphasized most was "relax," which he would draw out slowly to deliver his point.

The word got out in the little group of us who were studying with Dr. Wong that I was a dancer, and the students asked me if I would perform for them. I improvised a dance, after which the students applauded me enthusiastically. Our teacher just gazed at me for a few seconds in silence, then said one word, "Reeeelaxxxx." In my workshops, I often say this word in his style as an homage to one of my greatest teachers. This may, after all, sum up the most essential guidance most of us really need!

TAI CHI AS PRAYER

I studied Tai Chi Yang-style long-form, Qigong, and Tai Chi Sword religiously for two years—once a week for three hours each time. The rest of the week I practiced Tai Chi by myself, outside in a park or at the beach, for one hour every day, come rain or shine. I was living in San Francisco then, having moved there after graduating from UCI. Tai Chi became my salvation—my direct communion with the Beloved. Through its gentle, slow movements, I entered a silent conversation with life: with nature and the sky, with the visible and invisible worlds. It was profoundly healing. I had been shattered, and now I was being pieced back together again.

I experienced the universe as a vast womb—enveloping, embracing, and protecting me. My body seemed to expand to include everything around me: the clouds, the trees, the plants and flowers, the grass, the ocean, the birds. The whole Earth merged into oneness, and I was within that oneness. It was like praying again, much like the namaz (Muslim prayer) my grandmother taught me that I had stopped reciting years ago in Iran, after I had become alienated from it when the Islamic regime required all schools to enforce it as mandatory.

My dance training had begun in the element of fire, in yang—the masculine energy. Now I was entering the element of water, in yin—the feminine energy. Whereas flamenco is percussive and staccato, full of delineations and sudden shifts, Tai Chi flows continuously, without end. Through Tai Chi, you connect with the undercurrent of all movement: the profound, undifferentiated, dynamic stillness of the One. A deep calm arises from this great, peaceful energy of yin that underlies all things. In Tai Chi, the aim is to merge with this peace and let your movements grow from it in softness, in the way of the Feminine.

I had been shattered from climbing to the height of yang, and was now being embraced by the formless depth of yin—by non-being, the no-thing, or Hich, as we say in Persian. This is a concept cherished by Sufis who seek to be empty of their habitual self and filled with the Beloved. All my facades dissolved in the ocean. I no longer felt myself as a drop—I was the ocean. With flamenco, I was a drop, a diamond drop. Then I let go of even that and entered unknowing.

Like flamenco, Tai Chi offered me five profound initiations, in this case rooted in Taoist philosophy—gifts I now offer you that are equally resonant in dance and in life. These initiations flow through the very foundation of Dance of Oneness.

FIRST INITIATION: WE ARE EACH A RIVER

"The supreme good is like water, which nourishes all things without trying to. It is content with the low places that people disdain. Thus it is like the Tao."[1] For the Taoists, the concept of Tao, meaning "the Way," has two aspects: the Tao of transcendence, called Wu Wei, and the Tao of immanence, called Yu Wei or Tai Chi.

Tai Chi is a continuous flow that mirrors the qualities of water. It teaches us how to *be* rather than how to *know* or *do*. It shows us there is nowhere to reach, for we have already arrived simply by being fluidly present—flowing ever deeper into union with all that is. It asks nothing, claims nothing, and has nothing to prove. It is an unknowing, unassuming presence, a silent energetic conversation between our being and the greater whole—revealed as one and the same.

Our life's journey is the discovery of our own river's uniqueness, while remembering that we flow from the greater ocean and return to it. When we forget our source and rely only on our personal power, we become a whirlpool—cut off, circling in on ourselves. Eventually our river dries up, and we burn out. Then the ailments so prevalent today—depression, anxiety, and more—begin to set in. The river and ocean also remind us that, through Tai Chi, we can cultivate the capacity to flow like water and remain in motion, keeping pace with life's mutable, ever-changing nature.

This concept can also be understood in terms of energy and is closely linked to the new findings of physics, which we explored in chapter 2. Tai Chi teaches that that everything is energy, and that each of us is a unique manifestation of this one greater energy. We become cognizant of the greater energy by experiencing ourselves as boundless. It is from here that we can discover the unique, individual expression of the greater energy that we are. We don't create this energy; we need only to show up—relax, soften, and open—allowing ourselves to align with it so it can flow through us unobstructed, for the benefit of both the world and ourselves. In doing so, we shift from being a "whirlpool," closed in on ourselves, to allowing the "ever-flowing flood" to move us and flow through us—just as Rumi describes in the verses I shared in chapter 1:

You are water, but a whirlpool,
flow onto us and merge with us,
for we are the ever-flowing flood.[2]

SECOND INITIATION: MOVEMENT IS ALCHEMY

In Tai Chi, movement is used alchemically to create positive change in the physical body and its energetic system. The Taoist sages created a system to purify and transform matter into its most pure and radiant potential without the use of external agents. They developed exercises and meditations, including Tai Chi and Qigong, to circulate and gather what they called the "inner elixirs" of Jing (matter), Chi (energy), and Shen (spirit) at specific energy centers in the body. They called these main energy centers the three Dantians. The lower Dantian lies in the abdomen, the middle in the chest, and the higher in the head. Taoist sages understood the Dantians as crucibles or cauldrons of vital substance, energy, and awareness—vessels in which these forces are refined and transmuted to cultivate the fully realized, embodied human being.

THIRD INITIATION: THE UNIVERSE IS IN YOU

The third initiation builds upon the first two. Tai Chi teaches us to find the universe within, to recognize in our very body the evidence that all of life moves in patterns of energy—arising from the one great source and returning to it. We can expand ourselves energetically to embrace all of existence. The deeper we go inward, the more what we identify as "self" dissolves into the vast field of energy, merging with the greater whole.

The postures of Tai Chi are rounded, its movements circular and cyclical. The circle is a sacred form, inclusive and unifying. Rather than building barriers or wearing armor, Tai Chi shows us how to drop our resistances and melt away rigidity.

FOURTH INITIATION: MOVEMENT IS CONNECTION

Tai Chi calls us to practice movement as a way to connect with nature and all beings. It helps us cultivate a nurturing way to practice loving-kindness toward ourselves and all living beings. The movements literally caress and commune with the environment in long, flowing strokes, as every moment is savored and cherished as a sacred part of the journey.

Try this now: Let your arms rest by your sides. As you slowly lift them to shoulder level, allow yourself to luxuriate in each moment—as if this simple movement is a miracle. Sense the richness of your inner landscape and the environment around you.

It is especially powerful to practice Tai Chi in nature, where you can feel yourself woven into the web of life. Nature is spirit made manifest. Practicing in nature strengthens the lower Dantian, allowing you to absorb the Earth's energy and breathe in fresh—ideally clean—air. Once you have learned to conserve and circulate your own Chi, you can expand it by drawing from the inexhaustible reservoirs of Earth's Chi available in nature.

FIFTH INITIATION: FROM DUALITY TO ONENESS

Both the term "Tai Chi" and the symbol of the Tao exemplify the fifth initiation. Tai Chi, also referred to as Taiji, means flux, change, and the relationship between the opposing and complimentary forces of yin (the receptive, being, feminine, darkness, the formless) and yang (the active, doing, masculine, light, form). As noted earlier, Tai Chi is considered the Tao—the way of immanence—centered on dancing with duality, change, and constant flux. Tai Chi prepares us for the dynamic interplay between yin and yang that shapes all of life and guides us to unite these forces within ourselves and the world.

The yin/yang symbol of the Tao is one of the most beautiful representations of this idea. It shows the seed of yin within yang, and the seed of yang within yin. They are utterly inseparable. Not divided by a harsh, straight line but by a flowing curve, they continually flow into each other, become one another, and dance together while mysteriously retaining their own distinct function and identity.

CHINESE MEDICINE

The practice of Tai Chi fosters healing and equanimity, bringing balance to the body, being, and and environment. This is why it offers so many health benefits, including greater flexibility, strength, and cardiovascular vitality.

I was naturally led from Tai Chi and its healing powers to study Chinese medicine, which reveals the vital connection between movement and healing. This training taught me to both witness and experience the scientific as well as the therapeutic dimensions of movement. Yet the journey of acquiring this knowledge was intense and challenging.

DANCE YOUR LIFE

While I was still in college for Chinese medicine, all I wanted to do was dance and do Tai Chi, but I felt physically stuck, resentful of my rigorous studies. This inner conflict kept growing until it gave way to a realization. One day, when I was studying like crazy and complaining about the tedious intellectual world I had pushed myself into, I had an epiphany. I realized that I am a dancer, no matter what. I can dance regardless of the situation. I was dancing at that very moment! I was dancing the study of Chinese medicine.

The realization was liberating. I declared, "I am a dancer! Even if nobody else agrees, I'm still a dancer. I know I am a dancer." It was groundbreaking, filling me with both excitement and peace. It showed me that the dance never stops. Dance is not confined to the proscenium stage before an audience; it is woven into life itself. I had been initiated into being a "dancer of life." And I extend this invitation to you so you, too, can experience your life as a dance.

The invitation to dance onstage is only one kind of invitation. What about the invitation to dance your life? Dancing your life can bring joy, lightness, healing, grace, resiliency, adaptability, beauty, and creativity to any given situation. This attitude can transform what feels mundane, heavy, challenging, or difficult into opportunities for becoming whole. With this outlook and practicing Tai Chi daily, I danced through my studies and actually did quite well!

During this period, when I was very busy with exams, I once went five days without practicing Tai Chi, which was highly unusual for me. On the sixth day, I went to the park and began. I assumed the first posture but couldn't remember what came next. I started over again and again, but couldn't get past the opening posture. I was baffled. I had practiced Tai Chi every single day for five years, and after only five days, I had forgotten the sequence. How could this be possible? I froze in disbelief—until I heard a voice inside say, "You don't need to practice the form from A to Z anymore; this form is now who you *are*." This experience revealed that while it is essential to learn technique, once you have truly internalized it, you are free to express it in your own way.

I want to emphasize this point and remind you to freely express the material you learn in this book in your own unique way, once you have practiced and internalized it enough.

HEALING (NOT COMPETING) DANCE

In both flamenco and Tai Chi, there is a marriage of opposites. In flamenco, it is the union of rigor and surrender. In Tai Chi, it is the cultivation of infinite fluidity alongside a profound moment-to-moment self-awareness—a discipline of presence so finely tuned it feels like the opening of a flower.

I experienced yet another set of opposites when I entered my first year of graduate school in dance and choreography at UCLA. This was concurrent with my last year of training in Chinese medicine, when I was interning at the college clinic and seeing patients under supervision. Again, I found myself living in two worlds: the cutthroat, competitive world of dancers, where the limelight is rarely shared, and the world of medicine, where I was training to heal what was broken and fragmented.

Although it was often challenging to shift between the roles of dancer–choreographer and physician–healer, I believe the latter gave me a mind- and heart-set that ultimately saved me—both then and countless times since. When rivalry, jealousy, or suspicion—which can drown any performer, regardless of their talent and level of fame—threatened to engulf me, the attitude of physician/healer came to my rescue. This combination also gave rise to the healing dimensions in my dance modality. Medicine had trained me not to react with panic or defensiveness, but to diagnose the problem, seek its root cause, and work to heal what was fragmented and restore balance where there was discord.

For example, when I felt betrayed—by a colleague who copied my work without acknowledgment or a student who tried to teach Dance of Oneness without completing their studies—I turned to the methods of Chinese medicine. I traced the sense of betrayal back to its roots within myself, uncovering why it pierced me so deeply. In doing so, I began to transform the pain into deeper understanding and a renewed balance.

I had also worked to heal from the many painful episodes when, for example, I was invited to perform at a venue only to have the presenter change their mind and hire another artist—often someone who charged less. Instead of slipping into the standard mindset of performers, focused on scarcity and limited opportunity, I tried my best to think abundantly. I would remind myself: "There is room for all of us to shine. If I'm not performing this time, and so and so is, then this is how it was meant to be. I can accept it and allow others to shine. I don't always have to be the one in the limelight. The light can be shared and is meant to be shared. The more we share the light, the more we feel its radiance." I don't believe this attitude is prevalent in the professional dance world, and it has taken me considerable suffering and contemplation to cultivate it.

Life, like dance, is not about competition, but about healing, integration, and presence. By embracing opposites—rigor and surrender, discipline and fluidity—we can cultivate a mindset of abundance rather than scarcity. Instead of being consumed by jealousy or insecurity, we can learn to share the light and recognize that true greatness lies in inspiring others.

The cold, competitive atmosphere that permeates most dance classes never felt good to me. They breed insecurity and competitiveness. The two are inseparable. Competitiveness is born from insecurity, and insecurity breeds competitiveness. If each of us carried a healthy, loving sense of self, there would be space for all of us to coexist and express our brilliance. Establishing our individual worth and greatness should not depend on proving that we are *better* than others. Actually, our true greatness lies in how much we inspire others to feel their own worthiness.

A young, beautiful dancer once asked me a piercing question: "Why is it that most of the dancers I know who perform as bundles of joy and excitement, flying freely like birds onstage, are so miserable in their day-to-day lives offstage?" To me, the answer was obvious, though disturbing: A dancer who enthralls onstage yet is gripped with misery offstage leads two lives. In one life, she is the dancer who brings magic to audiences; in her other life, she doesn't know how to *dance* her life.

Perhaps very few dancers truly understand what it means to be a dancer—that dance is more than a vocation. Dance is a true spiritual path. The ultimate goal is to integrate the "dancer" and the person dancing and live one life. Any passion or vocation, when pursued deeply and authentically, can become such a path—a journey of self-discovery and alignment with our truest self, an opportunity to live with wholeness and purpose.

ACTIVE RELAXATION: BE YOURSELF (AND REMEMBER TO TRULY BE, YOU NEED TO NOT BE!)

Tai Chi teaches us to cultivate a calm and tranquil mind rooted in the present moment, moving and acting from a formless, receptive state—a kind of relaxed, non-doing doing. It invites us to focus the mind on the precise execution of each movement, anchoring our awareness in the now. This is presence without rigidity—what I call "soft precision."

The importance of maintaining a calm, relaxed attitude applies in all situations and shouldn't be confused with passivity, apathy, or lethargy. I call this "active relaxation"—the practice of remembering to release unnecessary tension, to not hold the muscles and flesh tightly. Active relaxation allows us to discover peace in nearly any circumstance. When we begin from peace, the actions that follow carry its energy and integrity.

You can say that active relaxation is the same as "being yourself"—accepting yourself as you are. When we embrace ourselves fully, we can relax, letting go of the anxiety born from striving to please others or to live up to imagined ideals impressed upon us by upbringing and life.

Yet, paradoxically, in order to truly *be*, we need to *not* be! Lao Tzu says, "All things are born of being; being is born of nonbeing."[3] This concept corresponds to the particle and wave theory in physics. You can think of being as particle or matter, and nonbeing as wave or energy. Since our bodies are actually 99.9999 percent space or energy, the greater part of us is actually in nonbeing—or what physics calls the vacuum (see chapter 2). As physicist Nassim Haramein writes,

> "Maybe instead of matter defining space, we should see space as defining matter. What's visible is not the whole of existence. The visible is really a small fraction of the large vacuum energy. The material world is a tiny dynamic of what is actually there."[4]

PRACTICE

BAPTISM BY LIVING WATER: ACTIVE RELAXATION
with audio component

This meditation invites you to soften, to release tension, and to rest in the living fullness of the present moment. Return to it whenever you feel called—especially when life feels heavy or your heart is unsettled.

You can do this practice following the Basic Meditation (chapter 4) or on its own.

Time required: 10–20 minutes

> Sit or stand with an upright yet relaxed posture. If you are seated, let your hands rest softly on your lap. Close your eyes and let your breath slow and deepen, flowing gently in and out of your nose.

> Envision yourself under a soothing and revitalizing waterfall—the living water of life itself. Feel this holy stream of love cascading

gently over your head, like a healing balm, flowing down the outside of your head and entering through your crown. Follow the pathway of this water as it moves on your skin and within you—down your ney, the reed flute of your body, along the chakras—baptizing, healing, and purifying you inside and out.

Feel the water softening the crown of your head, then gradually your face—temples, forehead, eyes, cheeks, jaw, and mouth. Let it wash and cleanse your thoughts.

Follow the pathway of the water into your throat, softening your neck and purifying your center of expression. Let it flow down to unburden your shoulders, then into your arms and hands, dissolving tension and healing any ailments.

Feel the water entering your chest—your heart center—melting tightness, washing away grief, and renewing your heart and lungs. Feel the living water of love flowing through your blood vessels, circulating throughout your whole body. Stay connected with your breath.

Allow the living water of love to move into your abdomen, softening any tightness, replenishing your organs, and revitalizing your Solar Plexus Chakra and sense of self.

Feel the water entering your hips, genitals, and sexual organs. Allow it to dissolve rigidity in your hips and awaken your creative center, renewing your connection to your sexuality and to the way you relate to others.

Follow the pathway of the water into your perineum, and flowing down your legs into your feet. Let it soften any tightness in these parts of your body. Feel the living water of love renewing your connection to the present moment and strengthening your bond with our Mother Earth—relaxing, nourishing, and healing you—letting "sickness blossom into health, and grief dissolve into delight," as Rumi says.[5]

Connect with the truth that your body is 70 percent or more water—the living water that carries wisdom and memory. Sense the river of your life flowing into the vast ocean. Dissolve the boundaries of your body into this greater ocean of love, the luminous field of energy surrounding you. Feel the bliss of surrender, the sweetness of being held, supported, and loved by the Beloved.

When you feel ready, draw in a deep breath, and as you exhale, gently open your eyes. Sense the subtle shift within you—the softening, the renewal—and welcome this state as a blessing to carry with you.

∞

You have been baptized by the living water of love into active relaxation and the fullness of the present moment. From this embodied place of ease, you are ready to continue integrating the first six rays of Dance of Oneness and to explore your inner world more deeply.

11

THE GURDJIEFF PROMISE

Presence in the Here and Now

Integration of Rays 1–6

Another modality that integrates the first six rays of Dance of Oneness—
and much more—is the Gurdjieff Work, also known as the Fourth Way.
This esoteric system of working on oneself, created by the influential spiritual teacher George Ivanovich Gurdjieff in the early to mid-twentieth
century, unites Eastern mysticism with Western science in service of
the harmonious development of humanity. It continues to be taught
in the Gurdjieff Foundation, an esoteric school with centers in many
cities around the world.

Just as I followed my passion for dance by diving into flamenco and
then Tai Chi, my passion for the Divine led me—at the age of twenty-two,
while deeply immersed in flamenco—to the Gurdjieff Work. Ever since
leaving Iran, I had been searching for the meaning of my life. I looked
into many different teachings and systems but couldn't really understand
them until I was led to the Gurdjieff Foundation and the book *In Search
of the Miraculous* by P. D. Ouspensky, which I found captivating. Not
only was the knowledge in this book conveyed in a way I could grasp, I
also felt I had been handed a clarifying lens through which to understand
the other spiritual texts I had previously read. My whole being ignited.
Once again, a rush of electricity surged through me, reminiscent of what
I had felt years earlier when I first read Rumi's words. I deeply resonated
with Gurdjieff's central premise—as elucidated by Russian philosopher

P. D. Ouspensky—that the human being is an unfinished creation, not yet the cosmically unique being whose intelligence and power of action mirror the energies of the source of life itself.

Gurdjieff maintained that human beings, as we are, are automatons—our thoughts, feelings, and actions little more than mechanical reactions to inner and outer stimuli. Unaware of this, we live in a self-deceptive state of waking sleep, imagining ourselves to be autonomous and conscious. In this sleep, Gurdjieff tells us, we are born, live, and die; we write books, invent religions, raise monuments, commit murders, and destroy all that is good.

BATTLE OF THE "I"S

Upon realizing we are all truly asleep, my first and foremost aim became to awaken! The fact that the teaching was centered around what Gurdjieff called "Sacred Movements" made his system even more intriguing for me.

After a trial period of several months—during which, in the tradition of esoteric schools, one's intent, devotion, and dedication are tested before being granted entry—I was admitted into the Foundation. There I became a fully committed seeker in the Gurdjieff Work, first in Los Angeles and later in San Francisco, for seven years.

I became more involved in the Work after my flamenco breakdown. The Work helped me see that the person called "Banafsheh Sayyad," whom I naturally referred to as "I," is not just one "I," but many, many "I"s, most of whom are in conflict with one another, mainly because of the absence of a single, cohesive "I." The catastrophic episode I had experienced with flamenco was a result of a battle between the different "I"s within me, each competing to rule the totality of me.

DO I REALLY EXIST?

Four years after I was first exposed to the Work, Southern California experienced the devastating 1994 Northridge earthquake near Los Angeles. As the first tremors struck, I rushed to the doorway of my family's home and sat on the threshold, the Earth surging beneath me in massive waves.

Faced with the possibility of imminent death, my whole life—along with all who were dearest to me—flashed before me. Yet a strange sensation overtook me: I saw the images, but I was absent from them. None of them seemed to matter—not my beloved family, not the man I loved, not even dance. The only moments that carried true weight, the only moments in which I felt I had truly existed, were those I had spent in the Work—even the initial trial period. These were the moments that possessed substance, that felt undeniably real. In that instant, I realized I was, in truth, only four years old.

Gurdjieff teaches that we have two births. The first is our birth into life. The second—by choice—is into consciousness: awakening from the "sleep" that is the prevailing state of humanity. Only after this second birth does our real life begin, and only then can we truly say, "*I am.*" At the time of the earthquake, I had been on the path toward awakening for four years. And I can say with certainty that even the smallest sincere act born of the wish to awaken from the illusion governing our lives is more real and life-affirming than all the relationships, ambitions, and possessions we imagine we cannot live without.

Human life in our modern era faces a grave crisis. One question arises before us: How can we reverse the process that seems to lead inevitably toward self-destruction? From what I learned in the Gurdjieff Work, our only salvation is to awaken, remember who we are, and become who we are meant to be in the service of Truth. Without this awakening and becoming, nothing else will save us. Only then can humanity free itself from the waking sleep that holds us in a hypnotic illusion.

In my time with the Gurdjieff Work, I was initiated into the path of awakening. From these initiations, I distilled five core teachings— offered here as the living architecture of Dance of Oneness.

FIRST INITIATION: PRESENCE BEGINS IN THE BODY

Just because we have a body does not mean we are present in it. I realized I was not consciously inhabiting my body, even after years of disciplined dance and movement. True presence in the body begins only when we recognize that, in our ordinary state, we are not actually living in the body—and when we commit to a disciplined intention to shift.

The Gurdjieff Work teaches us that the process of becoming conscious and present begins in the body. This is a law we cannot bypass as long as we are in a physical body. Our thoughts and emotions may drift into the past or fantasize about the future, but the body is always here, in the present. Thus, the gateway to presence opens by becoming present in the body. This is the ground of Dance of Oneness and its first ray. It is in this way that the Gurdjieff Work initiated me into both the earth and air elements, which is the domain of the mind.

At the heart of Gurdjieff's teaching is the struggle to be present in daily life—a struggle that opens us to full engagement with the duties and rewards of human existence here and now. Unlike many mystical paths that emphasize withdrawal from the world, Gurdjieff insisted that awakening and self-remembering must take place in the very midst of life. It is here, within the conditions of our everyday existence, that we remember who we are and what we are meant to become.

In the Gurdjieff Work, we are invited to face the naked truth of who we are—the brilliance and the bullshit alike. It is a call to be simultaneously noble and fully aware of your frailties and shadow. Once again, we encounter a union of opposites, a union grounded in humility: acknowledging your shadow while embracing your dignity as an embodied child of the Divine. The Gurdjieff Work offers a geometry of balance, helping us navigate between your creative and destructive sides and recognize them as two expressions of the same law.

SECOND INITIATION: INTEGRATION AWAKENS THE INNER MASTER

The only way to find balance is to avoid identifying with a single aspect of yourself. Can there be an authentic energy not dominated by one part or another? This is what you learn in the Work, leading to its second initiation: the recognition that wholeness and a true sense of self emerge only through the integration of the mind, body, and feeling centers. In our habitual waking-sleep state, these three centers function in isolation, each pretending to be the complete self, the "I."

According to the system Gurdjieff pioneered, the "work" we must do on ourselves engages body, mind, and feelings. When these three centers are integrated, they open the way for connection with soul and spirit. This parallels the Sufi understanding that fire—the symbol of spirit—arises only when earth, air, and water move together in harmony. In this analogy, the body is earth, the mind is air, and feelings flow as water.

In our ordinary state of waking sleep, we swing between "identifying" with one center and then another, which leaves us fragmented. At times, our centers even wage war against one another. The mind may insist on one thing while the feelings cry out for something else, leaving us unable to act. Such imbalance also manifests as one-sided development: people who are highly intellectual yet emotionally immature, or those with extraordinary control of the body but little development of mind or feeling.

After many years in the Work, I recall an intensive session at the Foundation that gave me a brief taste of what I could only call "integration." For a short period, I felt a balance among my three centers to the degree that I no longer identified with any one of them over the others, no matter the task at hand. I remember sitting in class at Chinese medical school, able to concentrate on the lesson, sense my body, and observe my shifting emotional responses to those around me—all without identifying with any single process.

I felt an inner freedom that allowed me to observe myself impartially in the midst of daily activities, with a spacious awareness in which experiences could arise without clinging or resistance. I perceived myself both from the outside, within the environment, and from the inside. I could focus on one thing while also hearing conversations in the room and sensing the larger field around me. I realized that as long as I remained unattached—regarding each sensation, thought, or event as neither greater nor lesser than another—I could sustain this liberated state. This perspective dissolved internal conflict and fostered integration. Nothing was rejected or overly emphasized, which opened into a more unified, whole experience of self. I was becoming attuned to my true nature.

This experience revealed that when we observe from both within and without, while remaining unattached, we align with our true self and open to an expansive awareness—no longer bound by fleeting identifications but embracing the fullness of being. The practice that most directly created this opening for me was the Sacred Movements.

Sacred Movements

The Gurdjieff Movements, which he encountered in part during his search in the monasteries and schools of Asia, are designed to unite mind, body, and feeling in the present moment. They cultivate the three centers simultaneously, creating conditions for inner freedom and an opening to the conscious energy of the true self. The dances involve intricate postures, sequences, and spatial patterns, always performed in groups. They are often accompanied by chanting or audible counting, which engages the mind; even a momentary lapse of attention can disrupt the entire group. The music, with its haunting rhythms and melodies, awakens the feeling center and opens the heart. The body is trained through the exacting execution of the movements, which require minute precision offered in harmony with an unceasing attunement to the greater whole.

All three faculties must be engaged in balance for the to be executed—let alone executed well! If the mind dominates—worrying about the next step, count, or chant—the rhythm falters. If one relies only on the body's memory or begins to "enjoy" the movements, one quickly falls out of sync with the group, the music, and the count. And if feelings take over, swept up by the beauty of the music, one may forget what comes next. Even for me, as a trained dancer, if I was not fully engaged, I would be thrown off immediately. Practicing this week after week honed my ability to divide my focus and remain present.

Consider what it means to cultivate undivided attention in your own life. This is not just about focusing harder, but about balancing all aspects of yourself—mind, body, and feeling—so no single part takes over at the expense of the others. The invitation is to be fully present, not in a passive way, but as an active participant in each moment, staying engaged without distraction and fostering a deeper connection to yourself and the world around you.

THIRD INITIATION: SACRED DANCE IS A SCIENCE

The postures and spatial patterns of the Gurdjieff Movements are rooted in sacred geometry and form a language that attunes both performers and audience to something impersonal, beyond subjective likes and dislikes—to the eternal ideals of Truth and Beauty. These ideals can be communicated only when dancers are wholly focused on embodying them through precise postures, sequences, and spatial designs.

In this way, the Gurdjieff Movements teach the very opposite of flamenco, where personal artistic expression is central. As Gurdjieff said, "Real art is knowledge, not talent."[1] Through the Movements, the dancer becomes an instrument of something greater, rather than striving for individual glory. This creates the possibility of trans-formation for both dancer and audience, as together they enter the universal field aligned with the eternal ideals of Truth and Beauty.

The concept of duende in flamenco is not so different from this. As I mentioned earlier, having duende means being overtaken by spirit. In flamenco, however, duende is revealed through the dancer's or musician's individual expression. In the Gurdjieff Movements, by contrast, the personal face dissolves into service of the greater. The aim is not to appear virtuosic or special, but to be available for a finer, freer energy to manifest through the integration of mind, body, and feeling in the present moment. It is about giving form to the laws of the universe through sacred geometric shapes. When a group dances with this shared intention—to serve the greater whole—they create an invisible sacred architecture that radiates harmony within them-selves, the group, and even the wider world. But when a dancer seeks to outshine the others, they separate themselves from the whole and disrupt the harmony.

The Gurdjieff Movements are about collective expression and par-ticipation in something larger, whereas flamenco is about individual creativity. Outwardly, the Movements are performed in public with the collective; inwardly, the practitioner remains unattached and free. Any attachment makes the Movements impossible to execute. Flamenco, by contrast, invites you to enter your attachments fully and burn through them. Both flamenco and the Gurdjieff Movements are alchemical and liberating, each in its own way making you a magician—free and unbounded, yet through different paths.

Group Synergy

I will never forget the first time I saw a live presentation of the Gurdjieff Movements. It was in San Francisco, during one of Gurdjieff's birthday celebrations, held annually on January 13 for the members of the Gurdjieff Foundation. The Movements were performed by two of the eldest groups, comprised of members who had been in the Work for at least twenty to thirty years, most of them in their sixties. In one particular dance, I saw the whole group move as a single organism with many faces. That vision of oneness left a profound impression on me. I saw how everyone was simply themselves, striving to integrate the three aspects of their being while moving in harmony with the whole. There was no showmanship, no attempt to dazzle with personal charisma—only sincerity and presence.

What I saw that night became engraved in me as a performer. Since then, I have instinctively strived to dance my authentic self, with no desire to impress. For me, being onstage is less about winning praise and more about whether I can be present and allow a finer energy to communicate through me for the benefit of all. What I am most wish to learn from my audience is what new insights and experiences they received—whether they could feel what I had been focusing on, channeling, or intending. This is what tells me how successful my performance was, and what I need to refine.

As you reflect on this, consider how it applies to your own life. The Gurdjieff Movements offer a path to transcend personal limitations by shifting focus from individual expression to a deeper collective harmony. Allow these ideas to inspire you to move beyond ego-driven desires and align with something greater than yourself. By integrating mind, body, and feeling with presence and purpose, you may discover a new kind of freedom—one that is not about standing out, but about becoming a conduit for higher awareness and unity.

FOURTH INITIATION: THE TRINITY

The fourth initiation opens to the Tao as a trinity. Rather than perceiving phenomena only as the play of dual forces, Gurdjieff reintroduced the ancient principle of the trinity as the foundational relationship of all existence. He called these forces the affirming, the denying, and the reconciling. You can picture the affirming force as yang, the denying as yin, and the reconciling as the circle that contains and harmonizes the two forces.

The principle of the trinity is reflected everywhere—even at the atomic level, where positive protons, negative electrons, and neutral neutrons form its structure. Trinity, as the intrinsic relationship underlying all that is, invites us to seek the third force whenever we encounter opposites. This third force is usually less apparent and less charged than the two opposing ones, yet it is essential: it connects and reconciles them. Forces such as consciousness and love—which are, in essence, one—belong to this third category. They are reconciling forces. They have no opposites.

FIFTH INITIATION: THE FOURTH WAY

The fifth initiation of the Work rests on what Gurdjieff defined as the Fourth Way. He claimed that all the traditional paths to spiritual enlightenment can be distilled into three: the Way of the Fakir, the Way of the Monk, and the Way of the Yogi.

In the Way of the Fakir, the seeker strives for self-mastery by struggling to control the physical body through difficult exercises and postures. In the Way of the Monk, the seeker pursues the same goal through the discipline of the heart, working to master feelings—akin to the Way of Faith, as practiced by Catholic monks, for example. In the Way of the Yogi, the seeker aims for mastery by working to control the mind, its habits, and its capacities.

Gurdjieff emphasized that while each of these paths aspires to develop a complete human being, each does so at the expense of other faculties. For this reason, he insisted on the need for a path that integrates and combines the three: what he called the "Fourth Way." Notably, the Fourth Way is fluid. It is not fixed or dogmatic, but draws from many teachings.

To walk the Fourth Way, as I do, is to remain open—willing to learn from everything and everyone without bias. It is to understand the essence of Rumi's words: "You will come to see that all evolves us."[2] When we cling to biases or judgments against people or things, we close ourselves to learning. Judgment ultimately shuts down the possibility of development. In the same spirit, Gurdjieff counseled: "Don't lie or steal, for you lie to yourself and steal from yourself."[3]

Consider how you might cultivate openness in your daily life. What does it mean to learn from everything and everyone? It begins with awareness—catching yourself in moments of judgment, questioning assumptions, and shifting from reaction to curiosity. When faced with a difficult person or situation, ask: "What can this teach me?" Rather than dismissing perspectives that challenge you, explore them. Observe your thoughts, emotions, and bodily responses without attachment, remembering that each moment is an invitation to grow. As you move through this book, I invite you to carry this openness with you—setting aside preconceptions, allowing the wisdom of many traditions to converge within, guiding you to evolve in unexpected ways.

PRACTICE

INQUIRY INTO PRESENCE
with audio component

This inquiry invites you to feel into whether you are truly present in your body.

Time required: 5–30 minutes

Sit in a way that feels comfortable, upright yet relaxed. Gently close your eyes and awaken the soles of your feet to the living ground beneath you.

Ask yourself:

Can I honestly say I am present in my body?

If so, what sensations, feelings, or awareness tell me I am present?

Whether your first response is "yes" or "no," enter the Basic Meditation practice (chapter 4). When you complete it, return to these same questions and notice if your answers have shifted.

∞

The forms and teachings we have explored thus far—flamenco, Tai Chi, and the Gurdjieff Work—embody the first six Dance of Oneness rays through their deep integration of presence, flow, and conscious embodiment. All three, especially the Gurdjieff Work, emphasize that "presence begins in the body" (ray 1). They also awaken us to "being a channel" (ray 2). Tai Chi does this by aligning with the flow of Chi, letting energy move effortlessly through the body; the Gurdjieff Work, by attuning us to what we serve; and flamenco, by inviting surrender, letting duende move through us.

Of the three, the Gurdjieff Work most powerfully supports the "journey in the upward spiral to become conscious" (ray 3) through sacred movements that heighten self-awareness and inner alignment. Each tradition teaches us to "ground ourselves lovingly in the Earth" (ray 4)—whether through the rooted postures and positions of flamenco and Tai Chi, or the Gurdjieff Movements' balance of stillness and motion.

The fifth ray—"embodying sexuality as the creative life force in the sacred union of polarities"—finds expression in flamenco's passion, Tai

Chi's harmonization of yin and yang, and the Gurdjieff Work's transformation of energy. Ultimately, all three paths nurture self-love and the capacity to move from our center (ray 6), guiding us to live from our essence with authenticity, grace, and conscious presence.

Having journeyed through the first six rays, we are now ready to move up to the seventh, which centers us in our heart.

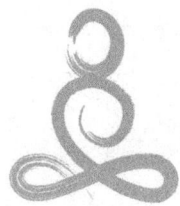

Chakra 4 of Union

Embody the Radiance and Wisdom of Your Heart

12

YOUR GALACTIC HEART

The Portal to the Infinite Field of Love

Ray 7: Let Your Heart, as the Portal to the Infinite Field of Love, Guide You

Chakra: 4—Anahata (Unstruck)

Location: Center of the chest

Anatomical areas of influence: Heart and circulatory system, lungs, shoulders, arms, and hands

Element: Air

Color: Green

The first six rays of Dance of Oneness have prepared us to now enter the domain of the heart, our portal to the infinite field of love. By awakening this center, we open to the vast intelligence that weaves through all of existence.

Let's begin by gently bringing your attention to your physical heart. Place one hand or both hands on the center of your chest, over your heart, and see if you can sense your heartbeat.

Your heart is roughly the size of a fist and sits in the middle of your chest, slightly to the left. It works every single second, twenty-four hours a day. In the course of one day, it beats over 100,000 times. In one year, your heart beats almost 38 million times, and by the time you are seventy years old, on average, it's made it to 2.5 billion beats. Not bad for a ten-ounce organ!

THE ALCHEMY OF THE HEART

Let's now tune into the mystery of how the heart works. Simply put, with each beat, the right chambers of your heart receive deoxygenated blood and send it to the lungs, where it is cleansed and infused with oxygen. At the same time, the left chambers receive this oxygen-rich blood and propel it through your body, delivering life to every cell. Within your heart, creative forces (oxygenated blood) and destructive ones (deoxygenated blood) coexist. Notice how the so-called destructive forces are always sent to the lungs to be transformed into creative ones. Imagine if your heart said, "I don't really like to deal with destructive forces. I only want to be around the creative ones. I'm not having a good day"—you wouldn't last long. If only our mind and emotions could truly understand and live the alchemy that is happening inside us all the time, we would be enlightened!

If your heart became sick and directed destructive forces back into your body, you would most likely die. You could say that this is what is afflicting our world. If we don't transform the bad blood and stagnant currents of our culture's toxic patterns, we will die out. We're being called to dance our lives in the same way the heart works—not to shy away from identifying what is destructive and does not serve the greater, but to recycle it, to transmute the dark into light on a consistent cyclical basis.

SPIRITUAL HEART

It is our spiritual heart that enables us to explore the shadow and uncover its treasures, allowing it to evolve us into wise messengers of love, under all circumstances. In some cultures, the physical heart and the spiritual heart are differentiated. In Persian, for example, the word for the physical heart is "ghalb," while the spiritual heart is referred to as "del."

In life, there's either love coming our way or a call to love. This means that either love is directly and unmistakably coming our way, or we need to find the depth and capacity within ourselves to recognize that whatever happens, however frightening or terrible, is a summons for us to love even more deeply and completely. This is the work of the carrier of light, the Darvish.

GUARDIAN OF LOVE

A lover is not made of confetti and romantic words in greeting cards. They grow out of the dung like a lotus flower and learn to bear everything. Can you be a lover in terrible times? This is perhaps the most important question in life. It's easy to be a lover when you're being shown love. But can you remember love in the face of hatred and antagonism? What does it mean to love even in the most dire circumstances and even when faced with evil? The message is hidden in the Persian word "mehr-ban," commonly used to mean "kindness," which, more precisely translated, means "guardian of love." Can you be a guardian of love—holding its expansive, boundless awareness—even in the face of what is difficult to love, without shutting down or contracting your heart?

THE POWER OF LOVE

Situated at the center, between the lower and upper chakras, the Heart Chakra mediates between body and soul, matter and spirit, physicality and energy, through love—the most powerful energy in the universe. In the Heart Chakra, we start to experience ourselves as more energy than matter, more wave than particle. The Heart Chakra, the domain of feelings, the center of tuning into the unlimited, is where we begin to experience this truth. Love is the doorway through which we experience the limitless.

Love is all there is, and in our essence, we are beings of love—radiant and whole in the unstruck, untouched, unharmed purity of our true nature, called Anahata in Sanskrit—the Heart Chakra. Yet through the ache of disappointment, the sting of loss, and the shadows of suffering, we built walls and armor around our hearts, forgetting the boundless love within. We are called to seek, find, and release these armors. Meanwhile, our physical heart works tirelessly with the lungs to transmute the dark into light, lovingly delivering to the body what is needed to sustain life.

THE HEART IS THE HOME OF THE BELOVED

In the Sufi path, the heart is considered the home of the Beloved. Since the Divine is infinite, the heart that is to be the home of the Divine needs to also be vast and infinite, capable of holding the whole. And what makes the heart vast is dancing with love, kindness, compassion, forgiveness, courage, and joy. We are called to polish our heart of the debris of forgetfulness, disbelief, doubt, and separateness, so the Beloved can reside at home.

HEART ARMOR

In Dance of Oneness, there are a number of dance and meditation practices designed to polish the heart and open the armor we wear around our chests so we can expand our heart to its true potential. The armor around the chest is formed by the fear of being hurt. Most, if not all, of us experience wounds of heartbreak, loss, and betrayal. These emotional catastrophes can constrict the heart and shut it down. We become mistrusting and suspicious and withhold love, not realizing that when we do this, we are, in essence, withholding our own capacity to become the abode of the Divine.

Rumi says, "The wound is the place where the light enters you."[1] He also says, "Pull the thorn of existence out of the heart! Fast! For when you do, you will see thousands of rose gardens blooming inside."[2] Heartbreak is meant to open us to the Beloved as the source of the one love. Our losses open us to that which is *never* lost: the presence of the Beloved—in our lives, and as our very being.

When we open ourselves to loving the Beloved as the source of the one love in everything that is, we begin to see our painful emotional experiences as portals to a greater love. Remember, as Rumi says, "Only from the heart can you touch the sky."[3]

HEART INQUIRY
with audio component

This inquiry invites you into greater intimacy with your heart. It can be done after the Basic Meditation (chapter 4) or on its own.

Time required: 5–10 minutes

> Sit comfortably, with an upright yet relaxed posture, in silence for at least a few minutes. Awaken the soles of your feet to the living Earth beneath you and place your hands gently on your heart center. Close your eyes and feel the rhythm of your heartbeat. Take a Love Breath.
>
> Ask yourself, and be present with what arises:
>
> How is this part of my body feeling right now?
>
> Can I rest here with ease?
>
> As I listen more deeply, what does my heart wish to share with me?
>
> What is love, as I experience it in this moment?

∞

THE LOVE FIELD

Our physical heart has an energy field that extends beyond it by about five to eight feet (two to three meters). Its electrical output is roughly sixty times stronger than that of the brain, and its electromagnetic field is about five thousand times greater. What we create in our heart field is broadcast outward, influencing ourselves and the world around us. The heart is literally an organ of perception and transmission.

Healing begins in the heart. Within our heart, there are some forty thousand specialized cells called sensory neurites. These cells function like brain cells, but they reside in the heart. They think, feel, and learn independently of the brain. Cardiologists often call this network "the brain in the heart." Remarkably, the brain receives many of its instructions from the heart—and those instructions are created by our own feelings, emotions, and beliefs.

According to the HeartMath Institute, the heart has the ability to think on its own, to remember and feel. Many signals from the body travel first to the heart before reaching the brain, where they significantly affect emotional processing and higher cognitive functions such as attention, perception, memory, and problem-solving. There is a constant conversation happening between the heart and the head.

When this communication is coherent, it triggers more than 1,300 beneficial biochemical reactions, including enhanced immunity, cardiovascular health, rejuvenation, and anti-aging effects. Positive feelings—such as appreciation, gratitude, care, compassion, and forgiveness—each a petal of the flower of love—establish this coherence, awakening what is known as the Heart-Head Union, or psychophysiological coherence.[4] This is profoundly important because the rhythm of a coherent heart is 0.1 hertz, the same frequency as the field lines of the Earth. When coherent, our heart aligns with the heartbeat of the Earth herself.

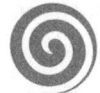

ROSE OF LIGHT
with audio component

This practice is designed to help you attune to your spiritual heart and enter into psychophysiological coherence, setting in motion a cascade of beneficial biochemical effects in your body that last for up to six hours. You may do this practice after the Basic Meditation (from chapter 4) or on its own.

Time required: 3–10 minutes

> Sit or stand with an upright yet relaxed posture. Feel Mother Earth lovingly through the soles of your feet. Come in touch with your breath, inhaling and exhaling deeply through your nose, and remember to stay attuned to this rhythm throughout the practice.
>
> Extend your right hand out in front of you, keeping your elbow slightly bent. Feel yourself holding in your hand the awareness of the heartbreak, horror, pain, and suffering in our world. Stay with this energy for about thirty seconds or so.
>
> Extend your left hand out in front of you, keeping your elbow slightly bent. Feel yourself holding in your hand the awareness of the beauty—around you, and within you. Feel the warmth, love, courage, and goodness in the people you know, and in yourself. Stay with this energy for about thirty seconds or so.
>
> Now, bring your hands together in front of your heart in a prayer position, holding both energies—the paradox of being alive in this wild, amazing, shattering, blessed mystery that is life.

Cross your hands on your heart. Close your eyes and sense the rhythm of your heartbeat, remembering with reverence how your heart miraculously holds both energies.

Bring your awareness to your breath. Inhale and exhale slowly through your nose, focusing on your heart. Breathe in and out of your heart space for about one minute. Feel yourself breathing in the precious life force and breathing out gratitude for being alive.

As you continue breathing in this way, visualize what you are grateful for, what you appreciate and love in this moment. You can imagine a loved one or a happy situation you have experienced. Keep visualizing this image as you breathe in and out of your heart space for about two minutes, feeling gratitude, appreciation, and love expanding within you.

Now, envision a rosebud at the center of your heart. This rose symbolizes your gratitude and love—your innermost essence, full of potential and beauty, waiting to unfold. With each breath, see the rose slowly blossoming, petal by petal, glowing with light.

As the rose begins to open in your heart, start moving your arms in slow, circular motions around your heart center with your eyes closed, nurturing the rose and gently fanning the petals open.

Synchronize your movement with your breath, feeling the rose expand with each inhalation as you extend your arms outward. With each exhalation, feel its light rooting into the Earth. Let the rose continue to grow in your heart space, radiating beyond—past the boundaries of your body.

Gradually, as the rose in your heart fully blooms, open your arms wide in a gesture of offering. Feel its radiance flowing outward through your chest and arms, filling the space around you with warmth and love. Sense a circle of light forming around you, as the love of your heart continues to shine forth.

Stay here as long as you wish, feeling the rose of light alive in your heart and transmitting it outward.

When you are ready to close the pracrtice, bring your hands back onto your heart. Reconnect with the living Earth through your feet, and return to the awareness of your physical body, traveling energetically upward from your feet to your crown. When you are ready, take a deep breath and, as you exhale, gently open your eyes.

Rub your hands together and lift your palms up in front of your face. Your heart meridian extends into your palms. Sense the warmth of your heart emanating from your palms onto your face.

Sit in stillness and just feel. Welcome the observations that emerge, and carry them with you. Throughout the day, tune into yourself and notice the subtle effects of this brief practice.

∞

In the journey of becoming fully human, it is essential to honor the primacy of the heart and to consciously awaken coherence. Every act of love, no matter how small, sends ripples outward, expanding the field of love in our world. Love nourishes health, stirs joy, and refines the gifts of the mind.

13

YOU ARE THE BELOVED'S BELOVED

The Ethereal Kiss of Persian Dance

Integration of Ray 7

Persian dance expresses the seventh ray of Dance of Oneness beautifully. The tender, sublime passion of this dance emanates from the soul of the rose, perfumed by great Iranian mystics like Rumi, fourteenth-century poet Hafez, and poet and theoretician Attar of Nishapur (c. 1145–1221). You can describe Persian dance as a rose opening with love for the Beloved—a melting and dissolving into subtle, tender ecstasy. It is a direct initiation from the Divine Feminine herself: Beauty pouring into you, awakening within you, and waiting to flower through you—a transmission of love that is ever-present, vibrant, and eternal. Persian dance is the manifestation of the Goddess in human form. It embodies the tender, sensual, and erotic—yet also the mystical, noble, and dignified—dimensions of the Divine Feminine.

When people ask me from whom I learned Persian dance, I always say, "From Persian music and poetry." It's difficult to tell which comes first—the dance, the music, or the poetry. I think of them as lovers and dance partners. The music taught me how to dance to it, merge with it, and resonate with its nuances and rhythms; the poetry gave me the inspiration.

I was inspired to uncover Persian dance from within myself, and the music and poetry became my guides. Having never seen any classical Persian dance performances in my formative years that inspired me, I had no teachers or mentors.

To clarify: "Persian" and "Iranian" are often used interchangeably. Iran, however, is home to many ethnic groups, with Persians being only one among them. In this chapter, my focus is on the style known as "Persian classical dance"—or simply "Persian dance"—which is distinct from the many regional Iranian folk and tribal dances, each with their own names and traditions.

PERSIAN DANCE

Persian dance has never been fully systematized, in part due to the repressive influence of conservative religious views in Iran. While Islamic Sharia law, consolidated in Iran by the 10th century, constrained cultural practices, it was particularly after the 1979 Iranian Revolution that strict interpretations of Sharia branded dance as haram (sinful). This led to the widespread suppression and marginalization of public dance, including Persian dance. Yet paradoxically, centuries of such suppression also created a kind of freedom: without rigid codification, the form has remained open to each choreographer's personal interpretation of the style.

Essentially, any improvised women's dance dating back to the Qajar Dynasty of Iran (1795–1925) referred to as Persian dance rests primarily on the dancer/choreographer's inspiration. Over time, the sources of inspiration have ranged from the fantastical imagery of Persian fairy tales in *One Thousand and One Nights* (compiled between the eighth and thirteenth centuries); to the refined elegance of Persian miniature painting, with its exquisite colors, balanced compositions, and meticulous attention to detail; to the lighthearted atmosphere of the harem (women's quarters) in the palace; and the vibrant culture of the bazaar, with its myriad stalls and shops found throughout the Middle East—to name only a few.

Regardless of the source of inspiration that shapes the content and intention of a choreography, certain shared characteristics often distinguish a dance as Persian. Most importantly, the dance closely mirrors the music. Much of its style and postures are drawn from depictions of women in Persian miniature paintings, especially the Saghi (winebearer and muse). In these paintings, the Saghi is sensual yet ethereal, dreamlike, with a fluid, flexible posture, often swooning as if intoxicated.

Similarly, in most Persian dance, the spine and upper limbs move with fluid grace, the movements executed in a lush, expansive manner with few sharp edges or staccato elements. The Saghi's world itself reflects this interconnected flow: an old man becomes a river, the river engenders a tree, the tree transforms into the Saghi, whose hair merges with the clouds in the sky. Everything blends into everything else— depicted as a true dance of oneness.

UNCOVERING PERSIAN DANCE

In my quest to know myself deeply, I became curious about my roots. I had unconsciously disassociated myself from my culture because of all the traumas I had experienced in connection to it. I believe it was necessary for me to disengage from the temporal aspect of my culture— namely the Islamic Revolution and its consequences—so as to discover its timeless beauty, which emerged for me through Persian dance and the Sufi path.

While I was studying Chinese medicine in San Francisco, I felt an overwhelming need to create dance. One day, I saw a flier for a dance festival seeking proposals. Visions of a mysterious Middle Eastern procession-like dance set to live music rose before my eyes, and I immediately sent in a proposal, which was accepted.

This moment marked the beginning of a new creative journey. Every morning, I awoke to a vast celestial music resonating from deep within. Was I hearing the music of the spheres? Its grandeur overwhelmed my senses, an ecstatic vibration beyond imagining, beyond description.

I have heard music on this scale a few times since. Once was during a tour with my dance company NAMAH, when we were waiting to board a plane at an airport. Sitting quietly, I suddenly began to hear a chorus of what I could only call angels singing very beautifully in total devotion in praise of the Divine. One of my company dancers brought me a cup of coffee, and I asked her, "Can you hear that? Can you hear the angels singing?" She looked at me quizzically and said it sounded like someone was vacuuming around the corner! Sure enough, there was—but in that moment, the vacuum's hum had opened a sonic doorway through which I could hear angels. The ordinary sound and the celestial singing became one, the machine itself opening my ears to the presence of angels.

Experiences like this attuned me to listen more deeply. Back in San Francisco, I woke up each morning to a different musical composition. I recorded what I heard by humming into a recording device so it could be recreated for the dance. On the bedroom wall by my pillow, I had placed an image of Saturn with its perfect rings, so it was the last image I would see before falling asleep and the first upon waking. I wasn't aware back then that astrologically, Saturn represents structure, definition, and limitation. This was exactly the influence I needed to create a dance from the uncharted territory of my psyche. In the evenings, I spent hours dancing to the music I had recorded until I was flat on my back with exhaustion.

OPENING

One late night in my apartment, when I had completely exhausted myself dancing to that morning's music, which had an Egyptian feel to it, I passed out on the sofa and fell into a reverie as the music continued to fill my ears. I'm not sure how much time passed, but all of a sudden, before my eyes arose a vision of the Great Pyramid of Giza, followed by the Sphinx. The Sphinx was so close and on such a grand scale, it filled my whole vision. I became terrified, and as I struggled to comprehend what was happening, the scene changed and the pyramid reappeared. I found myself in the position of the Sphinx on a conveyor belt with other people in the same position, traveling up the inside walls of the pyramid toward the top, which was open to the sky. I had a feeling that the pyramid was a portal to the stars. The vision was too much for me to bear, and I wished it would just go away.

There was nothing sinister or evil—it was simply the unknown, and I lacked the courage to enter. In the days that followed, the image of the Great Pyramid of Giza and the Sphinx would often rise up behind my immediate surroundings, so vast that people, buildings, and even mountains appeared like tiny specks in comparison.

I may not have been brave enough to surrender to this vision, but I did find the courage to choreograph and perform an original dance set to my own music inspired by ancient Egypt. I called the piece *Portal*, and it turned out to be a portal to the dance I yearned to express.

With this initiation, I felt the gates had opened for me. I had made my first public dance appearance after three years. The shame and guilt I felt about the destruction I believed I had caused in my flamenco days had kept me from dancing. But now, like the phoenix, I rose from the ashes and was recreating myself.

The mysterious vision and the music of the spheres were serendipitous signs heralding a new beginning, and I began to integrate the wisdom I had gathered over the past several years. I felt guided by my heart. When you allow your heart to lead, as the seventh ray of Dance of Oneness teaches, you become more attuned to serendipities and synchronicities. It is vital to listen to the whispers of the unseen as they flow through your heart.

Through *Portal*, Persian dance began to emerge out of the faceless flow of Tai Chi, the ferocity of flamenco, the objective precision of the Gurdjieff Movements, and the surrender of Sama (whirling). Inspired by the Gurdjieff Movements, I felt driven to communicate the sacred in dance, while also incorporating the sensual dimension I felt was missing in the Movements. Persian dance rose from the alchemy of the molten dark aspect of the Divine Feminine, the Tao, an objective approach to movement, and surrender—all channeled into the expression of a feminine lover in adoration of the Beloved.

I felt inspired by the ethereal, dreamlike quality of the Saghi—expressive of the air element. Having integrated fire, water, earth, and air to some degree, I now found myself guided more deeply into air. In dance, this element manifests as distant, unattainable, cool, lightweight, and celestial. Saghi is both the messenger and witness to love. By bearing the wine of love in the cup of her body, she also embodies not only love's devotion but also the intoxicating essence of wine itself.

POETRY IN MOTION

Rather than adhering to the prevalent versions of Persian dance I had seen—which struck me as too lighthearted—I sought to express mystical poetry and ancient myths and to evoke the shapes and forms found in Iranian calligraphy, architecture, and carpets. I began creating dances set to music with complex rhythms and slower tempos, which many considered unsuitable for dance. In short, I was being led to create dances never before seen—not by others, and not even by myself.

When you contemplate Iranian culture, you encounter subtlety, nobility, and refinement. These qualities shine through the language, poetry, literature, philosophy, music and instruments, architecture, carpets, calligraphy, cuisine, and more. All express the lover's radiant love and adab for the Beloved, as well as a noble commitment to making life transcendentally beautiful—which it already is, as the creation of the Beloved. Even the very notion of "paradise" originates from the Persian word "parādaiĵah," later becoming "pardis" (from the Avestan "pairi-daêza"). One could say that no other culture has woven a language around love as profoundly as the Iranians.

To communicate the soul of Iran, I was guided to collaborate with my sister Maryam in converting the Persian alphabet into postures. Joined together, these postures enabled us to dance words like "eshgh" (love) and verses of poetry by poets like Rumi. I now had a system in which choreography did not arise from my personal direction alone, but allowed a transmission to move through me. To me, dance is a kind of calligraphy, and calligraphy is a dance—and with this technique, I began to literally unite the two.

Since light is the basic building block of all that exists, movement can be seen as calligraphy drawn in light across space. Reality itself becomes divine calligraphy. By dancing the alphabet, we become the Divine's brush, inscribing radiant letters into space and weaving poetry into motion.

DANCING FOR THE BELOVED

When Persian dance awakened in me, I began to dance for the beloved I had lost in my early twenties. I envisioned him as I moved—my love flowing toward him, my grief for his absence woven into every gesture. In the dance, I adored and enticed him, I surrendered and seduced him, but most of all, I longed for him.

Longing and adoration are at the heart of the Iranian soul—a longing for primordial union with the Divine: an intimacy once known, then lost, yet forever sought in the yearning for reunion. Rumi opens his masterpiece, *Masnavi*, with these timeless words: "Listen to the reed's lament, as it recounts the tale of separation."[1]

I shaped my vision of Persian dance through a tantric longing and adoration of the human beloved. In this dance, you envision the beloved you are dancing for and feel them awaken in the minutest fibers of your body, soul, mind, and feelings. I danced for my imagined human beloved until he slowly dissolved into the Divine Beloved, and I found myself dancing for the Beloved who is *everything*—both within me and beyond. That tantric experience of ecstatically adoring and longing for the man I had lost became a doorway into the mystery of my soul's yearning for union with the One. To adore is to find "a door." It was essential to begin with the human beloved, as the ambassador of the Divine Beloved. This experience revealed to me that all loves are but rays of the one and only love—the love of the Beloved.

APHRODITE-ANAHITA APPEARS

When the Beloved emerged, my whole being transformed into Aphrodite-Anahita and received Him. I was baptized in the honey-eyed waters of the Goddess herself. Persian dance became the liberation of Aphrodite-Anahita within me. For Iranians, the qualities associated with the Greek Goddess Aphrodite—love, beauty, fertility, and sensuality—find their parallel in the ancient Persian Goddess Anahita. Revered as the divinity of water, healing, fertility, and wisdom, Anahita embodies both the nurturing and the fiercely powerful aspects of the feminine. Her connection to water symbolizes purification, life-giving power, and the flowing grace of wisdom and memory, making her a deeply venerated figure in pre-Islamic Iran.

In my dance, the Beautiful One—she whose ageless sensuality and fertile presence compel the whole world to melt in adoration—emerged from under the veil. In myth, it is said that with each step she took, flowers blossomed beneath her feet. Animals who beheld her were overcome with desire and rushed away to mate. Everywhere, Eros was awakened.

In the beginning, she was shy within me—veiled, demure, more pious than sensual—yet slowly relaxing into herself. I was on a journey of healing, piecing myself back together from fragmentation, having lived, like so many of us, in the chasm between the sacred and the sensual. Through Persian dance, my sensuality—and indeed my femininity—was being sanctified, though this awakening did not happen overnight. In those early days, my devotion was directed mainly toward uncovering the sacred dances that may once have flourished in pre-Islamic Iran.

I wanted to uncover the earliest remnants of my culture, but didn't find any historical accounts of dance. I began to create movements and sequences by meditating on hymns and from my own imagination. I looked to ancient reliefs and artifacts for inspiration. I created very angular, ritualistic movements inspired by fire, depicting carriers of the flame. Originating in ancient Iran, the Mehri or Mithraic tradition, which centers around the solar deity Mehr (associated with the sun, love, and friendship), awakens us to our essential spark that can become ablaze through cultivating inner strength and moral clarity.

With this arsenal of new movement, which I called "Contemporary Mystical Persian" dance, I began performing more and more after my three-year hiatus. Together with a dear friend and colleague, I created the dance ensemble NAMAH. "Namah" in Avestan means "reverence, greeting," and "prayer." It is also the root of the Sanskrit word namaste—literally "I bow to you," and poetically understood as "the light within me salutes the light within you." From the same root comes "namaz," the Arabic word for "prayer." Namah perfectly expresses my aim in dance: prayer, devotion, and honoring both one-self and all beings as divine.

DANCE AS THE BELOVED'S BELOVED
with audio component

Persian dance taught me that just as the Divine is my Beloved, I am also the beloved of the Divine. Unless I recognize myself as the beloved of the Beloved, the love affair remains one-sided—yet this can never be, for as Rumi reminds us, "What you seek is seeking you."[2]

In this practice, I invite you to envision yourself dancing for the Beloved, as the Beloved's own beloved.

Time required: 5–15 minutes

> Select a piece of music that awakens your sensuality. Wear flowy attire that lets you feel both free and sensual.
>
> Begin in stillness with an invocation to the Beloved, letting words flow spontaneously from your heart. Speak directly to the Beloved, knowing you are being heard and received.
>
> As you start to move, imagine the Beloved watching you. Pour your adoration into each gesture, and at the same time, feel yourself adored in return—recognized as the beloved of the Beloved.
>
> When your dance naturally comes to a close, settle into stillness, as if held by the Beloved. Let the resonance of your movement shimmer within you. Sense the aliveness in your body, feel the emotions awakened, and savor the sweetness of

being the Beloved's beloved. Allow this stillness to be as sacred as the dance itself.

Give yourself a quiet moment to let your experience flow onto the page.

∞

Persian dance, with its grace and devotion to love, invites us to step through the portal of the heart into the infinite field of love. It is a dance of body and soul. When we surrender to the heart's rhythm, love streams through us, weaving harmony between inner and outer worlds. Moving from the heart, we enter the rhythm of the infinite love that animates existence.

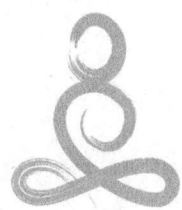

Activate Chakras 5–8

Awaken the Transformative Energy of Your Spiritual Centers

14

LET YOURSELF
BE DANCED

Trance and the Ecstatic Presence

*Ray 8: Let Go of Your Thinking and
Allow Yourself to Be Danced*

Chakra: 5—Vishuddha (Purified)

Location: Throat

Anatomical areas of influence: Throat, neck, thyroid,
parathyroid, jaw, mouth, ears

Element: Sound

Color: Turquoise

Journeying upward from the Heart Chakra to the Throat Chakra, the
eighth ray invites you to release attachments to your body, mind, emotions, and concepts, and to surrender instead to the pure flow of the
dance. In this trance-like state of being moved by something greater than
yourself, you step into ecstatic presence, where the boundaries of self
dissolve and you merge with the infinite rhythm of the universe.

Situated between the head and the heart, the Throat Chakra serves as a bridge between the two, giving voice to the truth of the heart while fostering coherence and union with the head. It is the center of willpower, choice, expression, communication, and discernment, and connected to your voice. This chakra relates to your ability to speak your truth and to express your ideas clearly, truthfully, and gracefully—attuning in harmony with both inner and outer vibrations.

We are living through a Throat Chakra crisis across much of the world—an era of deception and outright lies, where truth is blurred and misinformation spreads widely. So how do we decipher what is true in this kind of climate? We listen to the depths of our heart, to the still, small voice that whispers within.

One of the heaviest armors we wear—especially as women—rests around the throat and neck. This armor is forged from withholding truth and from the inability to express our authentic self. Many of us carry both personal and collective wounds: the trauma of being silenced, stifled, and oppressed. In far too many places, the old belief still lingers that "a good woman should be seen but not heard." And in some places, like Afghanistan, she is not even allowed to be seen.

ALIGN WITH TRUTH

The Throat Chakra is our center of will. In the Solar Plexus Chakra, we cultivate willpower and self-authority, yet true authority arises only when we align ourselves with divine will—with a power greater than our own—bringing what we desire into harmony with what life desires from us.

The invitation of the Throat Chakra, echoed by the eighth ray, is to release what we think we know and align with divine will—divine truth. In the ancient Iranian tradition, one of the names of the Divine is Raasti (Truth). To align with truth and trust in the greater design—not from fear, but by choosing love—lies at the heart of the Sufi path and finds exquisite expression in Sama.

In dance, we control our turns; in whirling, we surrender control and allow the spin to carry us. Most of us love to spin as children, but abandon it as we grow older. I never stopped. I relished the euphoria it gave me—you might even say I was a little obsessed.

Around the age of twenty-two, without any apparent reason, I began to whirl for long stretches of time at night, in complete darkness and silence. Yet inside me there was only noise—the ceaseless chatter of my mind, which grew louder and more absurd the longer I whirled. Still, my intention was to persevere: to keep whirling, no matter what.

THE ENEMY INSIDE

As I whirled, a cacophony of voices erupted in my head—voices I hadn't even known were there. Looking back, I can say it was my ego, appearing in a myriad of guises. It shifted from mocking me to outright terrorizing me. More than once I stood on the brink of freezing in fear: "Oh no, someone has broken into the apartment," my ego warned, "he's here to kill you—you must stop to save yourself!" Yet something deeper in me knew I had to keep turning, and I did. My ego also preyed on any discomfort in my body to halt me: "My ankle hurts. I should stop." And on and on it went. Years later, I read in *A Course in Miracles* that the ego is the part of us that hates us, the part that insists on maintaining a chasm between the self and the Divine—no matter the agony it causes. This struck me deeply; I had firsthand experience.

My early experience of whirling was like an exorcism—a fierce clearing and a realignment with my essence. It took three or four sessions, each lasting several hours, before I began to taste fleeting intervals of silence in my mind. Each time I set out, I faced a new uphill battle with my ego. Yet by the end of each session, those brief moments of stillness and expansive emptiness were a glory unlike anything I had ever known.

After whirling, I often experienced visions beyond words. On one occasion, when I stopped, I saw myself as a translucent, three-dimensional, violet-hued diamond turning amidst an infinite constellation of rotating diamonds in every color, all arrayed in a grid stretching endlessly in every direction.

The more I whirled, the clearer, more lucid, and freer I felt. The fog of forgetfulness and sleep gradually lifted from my eyes, and I felt myself slowly being cleansed of my "self." Whirling had become my prayer and my communion with the Divine, who felt more and more like my Beloved.

THE NAMELESS IS MY BELOVED

This was by no means a straightforward scenario though. Once again, I felt myself living in two worlds. In one, I was cultivating an intimate relationship with the Unknown as my Beloved through whirling. In the other—the world of the Gurdjieff Work—any name or reference to the Unknown was met with scrutiny.

In the Work, you learn that one essential difference between religious institutions and spiritual paths is that religion provides answers, while true spiritual work offers only questions. We acquire our beliefs and habits in the state of waking-sleep, and these very beliefs and habits keep us imprisoned in that state. Part of me was one with the Beloved; another part of me questioned the validity of that part. In short, I had no peace. Was it wiser to stop pursuing both worlds at the same time and just immerse myself in one? If so, which one?

MEVLEVI SAMA PRESENTATION

I was still wrestling with this inner conflict when I learned that a group called the Mevlevi Order of San Francisco—a Sufi order devoted to the tradition of whirling—was about to present a public Sama. I had never before witnessed a complete whirling ceremony.

The evening opened with a brief introduction inviting us to release the idea that we were merely spectators and instead to see ourselves as inwardly participating in the journey. I felt a rush of excitement and curiosity, anticipating what I believed to be the aim of the whirling ceremony: to mirror the cosmic order—the planets circling the sun, all revolving around the center. I wondered how such a vast vision could ever be conveyed through dance.

The venue was a high school basketball court, with the audience seated on bleachers. The performers—men and women ranging in age from thirty to eighty, dressed in black robes and tall hats—entered the court. The musicians began to play, and the whirling commenced.

At first, I was taken aback. Most of them were not technically proficient, and some stumbled quite frequently. They didn't turn in unison or even at the same tempo. Each seemed to turn from their own inner impulse. In flamenco ensemble dances and in the Gurdjieff Movements, I had been taught to move with the tempo of the music, expressing it with precision and in harmonious unison with the group. Anything less was considered sloppy and unacceptable.

I immediately became very critical. As I became more and more identified with my own mental chatter and disconnected from what I was witnessing, I remembered the invitation I heard at the onset of the ceremony to "participate inwardly." This very question created an opening—a possibility to think differently. Could it be that I also played a creative role in what I wished the ceremony to be? Was it possible that I was contributing to the harmony, or lack thereof, with my thoughts? Precisely at that moment, I caught sight of an elderly man, whose orbit had brought him to my side of the court. He whirled with such grace and symmetry that I was moved to tears. His movements illuminated the music with a depth I could not describe. To me, his whirling was even more sublime than the music itself.

In his face, I caught a glimpse of the Beloved, for *he* was gazing at the Beloved. Looking at him, I felt myself gazing at the Beloved too. This was not an ordinary performance; it was a transmission that forever shaped my dance.

For a long time, my eyes followed the man wherever he whirled. Then I began to look at other whirlers. I saw them differently now. I looked at them with compassion. I was touched by their courage, which allowed them to whirl despite physical restriction and imperfection. I asked myself, "What is perfection after all? Is it found in form and flawless execution, or does it also live in our dedication and purpose—in the act of giving our best despite our limitations?" Something shifted inside me around the question of perfection. The ceremony had given me a profound revelation. I left the gym elated and deeply grateful.

I walked to my car and was stunned once again! Earlier that day, I had filled my car to capacity with items to be delivered to the Gurdjieff Work house. When I emerged from the performance, I found every door and the trunk flung wide open. The windshield wipers were pointing outward like the arms of whirlers. And still—not a single item was missing.

What could this mean? I stood amazed. It felt as though the doors of my psyche had been thrown open, inviting me into the mystery, yet fully protected. In that instant, my two divergent worlds merged into one beyond conception, and all I could do was whirl—right there on the street, on a chilly yet vibrant San Francisco evening.

Let this story invite you to move beyond passive observation and engage with life from within, knowing you are the co-creator of all you witness and experience. True perfection isn't in flawless execution, but in presence, devotion, and courage. Just as my car's open doors mirrored my own inner opening, life constantly offers us symbols and synchronicities that guide us beyond rigid dualities. When we release judgment and enter into presence—which is the invitation of the eighth ray—we step beyond dualities into the mystery of life and align with a deeper flow, one that invites us to trust, embrace the mystery, and recognize the unseen forces supporting our journey.

THE MEVLEVIS

The word "Mevlevi" is the Turkish pronunciation of "Mowlavi," which is Rumi's pseudonym in Persian, meaning "master." The Mevlevi Order was established in Turkey by Rumi's first son, Sultan Valad, after his death. Rumi—a Fourth Way teacher in essence—did not believe in institutionalizing spirituality, though he emphasized the importance of learning from teachers when embarking on a spiritual path.

The orders in the Sufi tradition are named after great sheikhs (teachers) who transmit teachings to their followers and students. In some Iranian mystical circles, the name "Sufi" is considered derogatory, used to describe someone pretending to possess spiritual knowledge or power. Both Rumi and Hafez warn of such charlatans on the path—those who profess to be Sufis but are so only in appearance. Some adopt the outer signs of Sufism—its robes, language, and postures—in order to gain authority, influence or material advantage. Others may fool themselves, mistaking secondhand knowledge and rehearsed gestures for genuine awakening. In both cases, the essence of the path is lost, for true Sufism is not in appearance but in inner transformation.

My father told me stories about his own father—a well-known Sufi in his own time—who would take him to their gatherings when he was a child. My grandfather—peace be upon him—had been given the venerable title of Shah (King). I never got a chance to speak to him about the order he belonged to because he passed away when I was nine years old, before I became aware of the Sufis.

In the Sufi path, regardless of the order, Sama is a central practice. Remember that "Sama" in Arabic means "to listen." The whirling of the Mevlevi Sufis is a form of Sama. It is based in Rumi's passion for whirling, which was central to his life and teaching.

SAMA OF SOUL AND BODY

The invitation in Sama is to let stillness be your anchor and center of gravity, so that all else unifies around it and its radiance fills your whole body and being—becoming ever more integral to the awareness of who you are. Sama combines a foundation of silence with ecstatic heart-opening through music and dance.

In Sama, you can experience the infinite within the finite space of your body. Once during a Sama, as I was holding my right hand up, I literally felt wine pouring into my hand and into my arm. It came into my heart and saturated my whole body. It was real; I could taste it and feel its wetness. The wine is not of our making. Our task is to become a chalice that can hold the wine of divine grace and to serve it to others.

SUFI TRAINING

Shortly after relocating to Los Angeles to pursue my graduate work in dance and choreography at UCLA, my search led me to the Nimatullahi Sufi Order, which I was invited to join after attending a few public sessions. Spoken language played a very small part. In each session, there was a brief discourse on a Sufi theme, but the essence of the teachings was transmitted through music and poetry, often performed live.

As the music began—often lasting for hours in complete darkness—the saalek (seeker of truth, a reference to seekers on the Sufi path) was encouraged to enter into Sama, which in this case meant seated meditation. The music would always begin slowly and gradually accelerate, becoming more and more exuberant, until it carried the saalek into ecstasy.

This form of meditation was profoundly different from what I had known in the Gurdjieff Work, where we often began with a short guided journey led by an elder, followed by complete silence. Most of the time during those sittings, our eyes were closed. But on occasion, after an intensive three-day period, we would sit together in meditation with our eyes open. These moments were truly remarkable: I would not become distracted at all and could sustain a sense of balance and order between inner stillness and outer perception.

In the Nimatullahi Tarighat (path), the way we reached balance and a sense of order was different: the music itself became our guide. Often repetitive, it was played on a string or woodwind instrument, accompanied by the daf—a large frame drum with chains along its inner rim, central to many Sufi rituals in Iran and beyond. I have always felt a profound connection with the daf; its ancestral sound can draw me into trance almost instantly.

WHAT IS TRANCE?

The more we let go and surrendered, the more the music and poetry entered our bodies, drawing us into trance. At times, people would cry out or shriek in ecstasy, as if being purged of what was not truly their essence. At first the movement is chaotic, but within the chaos harmony emerges, and the body begins to move with symmetry and order. I witnessed this in others and experienced it in myself extensively. This order does not come from us; it moves through us. Its emergence signals that we have been cleansed of impurities—emotional, mental, or physical—accumulations of unresolved issues that keep us from wholeness and from living in our essence. These accumulations must be purged from time to time, or they harden into disease.

In many traditions, trance ceremonies create conditions for purging impurities—both in their early stages and later, when they may have hardened into ailments or even disease. In Dance of Oneness, we always devote generous time to shaking and purification, what I call "dusting ourselves." This practice helps clear away the debris that accumulates in body, heart, and mind through the currents of life.

ECSTASY MEANS BE HERE NOW

Trance and purging lead to ecstasy. "Ecstasy" means "to be present in the moment." Remember how the Persian language reflects this very clearly. The word "haal" in Persian means both "ecstasy" and "the present moment." What I had come to know as presence through the Gurdjieff Work was undergoing a great transformation. The knowledge I had acquired with my mind in the Work was now descending into my heart.

My body had been prepared for this meeting. From the Gurdjieff Work, I had learned the importance of embodiment and sober clarity; now I was uniting body and mind with heart and ecstasy.

The main hall of our khaneghah (Sufi temple) was very welcoming, warm, and cozy, with traditional Iranian decor, much like my grandparents' home in Iran. Filled with colorful rugs and big pillows against the walls, and adorned with paintings, poetry, calligraphy, and various gems and jewels, it felt like one big heart to me.

For a time, as I drove or walked through the streets of Los Angeles, I experienced entire avenues, buildings, and cityscapes as if they were arising from that main hall. All of it seemed contained within the walls of that special, cozy room where, like the heart, everyone was free to be themselves. My sister also attended the gatherings with me, and when I shared my vision of the city held within the walls of the khaneghah, she told me she had been seeing the very same thing.

Traditionally, a khaneghah is a place where all are welcome and the door is always open. It is here that one learns to become a Darvish—a person known to everyone as a true friend, who makes no distinction between kin and stranger. Sufis often refer to the Divine as the Friend, and the Darvish, as a friend of the Friend, lives this friendship with the Divine through their interactions with all people and creatures. All relationships flow from this one relationship. A Darvish is a friend to everyone, meeting each person exactly where they are. They don't share the secrets of the heart with those who do not live from the heart. Rumi says, "Beloved, your love has transformed me. I am alive with your living and dead with your dead."[1] In other words, "I am alive with those who live in you, and dead with the ones who are dead to you," meaning as a friend, I simply mirror each person's essence back to them.

THE QADERI SUFIS

I started the graduate program in dance and choreography at UCLA around the same time I entered the Nimatullahi Tarighat. I don't think I could have withstood the challenges of my studies had I not been in the Tarighat, where I experienced the continual cycle of death and renewal through trance. During this time, I also became acquainted with the trance practices of another Sufi Tarighat, the Qaderi, through a friend who had filmed them in their home region of Kurdistan.[2]

Watching the ceremony of the Qaderi of Kurdistan on film was nothing short of an epiphany. It begins with the saalek seated on the ground, chanting the names of the Divine in remembrance (zikr) to a slow rhythm on the daf and other percussive instruments. Gradually, as the tempo accelerates and the chanting and drumming intensify, the saalek rise to their feet and, with arms interlinked, begin to bow their heads forward and backward in unison. The bowing deepens with the music until their whole spine is moving with it. Their long, flowing hair, once tied back or hidden beneath a hat, is loosened and cascades up and down with the rhythm of their movement.

Their ages range from late-teens to nineties. Their different hair color—some black, some silver—lashes forward and back to the beat of intense drumming and chanting, unleashing a tremendous power that evokes the image of oceanic waves rising and receding in cycles of death and rebirth. The group moves together toward a unified trance, while some saalek, guided differently by spirit, break away to whirl or move in other trancelike ways.

Often, someone from the outside community who is facing mental or emotional challenges is placed at the center of the hall where the ceremony unfolds. The high vibration of the music, chanting, and trance movements is said to draw the ailment out of the person. Gradually the ceremony swells, rising to a pinnacle of embodied grace, where it lingers for a time before slowly tapering down.

When I watched the footage of the Qaderi Darvishes, I felt a deep ancestral connection. It was like my first encounters with flamenco and Tai Chi—not simply recognizing the movement, but feeling I had moved in that way before, as if it were utterly natural to me. I saw the Qaderi as part of my lineage and longed to return to Iran to participate in their ceremonies. But this was not possible: because of my father's name and his political activities against the Islamic Republic, I could not return. My family had been granted political asylum in the United States on the grounds that we would face persecution if we went back. So I connected with the Qaderi energetically, from afar.

THE ART OF FALLING

I listened to the Qaderi recordings and journeyed deeply with their music through whirling and the movement inspired by them. Many times, I whirled so fast and intensely—and fell to the ground so hard—that I feared every bone in my body was broken, only to discover I wasn't even bruised or scraped! The way our bodies are protected and safe-guarded in these journeys is nothing short of miraculous. I came to understand that every time I fell, it was because I was trying to break through to a new level of being for which I was not yet ready. Falling was the natural consequence of utterly letting go. In those journeys, I had no desire to ground myself; I longed only to fly into the vast unknown. I would encounter dimensions within me that I was not yet able to inhabit, but for which I was being prepared. Falling, I learned, can sometimes save you from pushing too far too fast—and from losing yourself.

THE QADERIS IN MADRID

While on tour in Europe for performances and workshops, I received word that the Qaderi had arrived in Madrid, where I was, and were scheduled to perform at a theater outside the city. I was overjoyed.

Seven men with long silver hair—including the esteemed Sheikh Mirza Agha Ghosi, their elder and teacher who passed away not long after—peace be upon him—took the stage. The sheikh chanted and played daf with three of the men, while the other three men did the reverential bowing. Though their performance was not perfect in technique, right from the very beginning, all seven moved as one. From the first note to the last, I felt waves from an ancient ocean rise through them and pour over the audience like a blessing. These waves swept over me and carried me to a point where I could not feel the ground anymore.

When the program ended, I felt I was no longer in my body. After I got ahold of myself a bit, I walked backstage to see the sheikh.

There he was, seated in the middle of the hallway leading to the dressing rooms. His presence radiated magnificence and power. I stood before him in silence, and we looked at one another without a single word—yet in complete communication. I cannot fully put into words what was transmitted to me that evening, only that it had to do with what Sufis call Vahdat-e Vojood—the unified field of being. Though I may never be able to fully describe that experience, it has profoundly shaped me and my dance.

THE LANGUAGE OF TRANCE

The movements I have introduced you to—flamenco, Tai Chi, the Gurdjieff Movements, Sama, Persian dance, and trance—all emphasize the eighth ray of letting go and being moved by something greater, whether we call it duende, the Tao, consciousness, or the Beloved. Through this surrender and openness, I invite you to be passionate about the dance and to let it move you completely. And I know this because, for me, if I am only dancing my own dance, it soon becomes boring. I long for freshness and the unexpected. I yearn for a love-making to take place inside me—between spirit and matter, body and soul.

I had begun my journey in creating a new expression in Persian dance and came to an impasse. I didn't want to simply direct the dance; I longed *to be danced*. So I abandoned myself to trance, and it wasn't until I had let go of my knowing that all my learning became integrated into what later came to be Dance of Oneness.

As alluring as the power of the Divine Feminine was, as profound as my devotion and adoration to a Beloved I thought I knew felt, and as essential as the Tao and science seemed, I made a conscious choice to embrace the unknown. Once I fully surrendered to not knowing, everything I thought I knew began to serve what I did not know.

This is how I uncovered my form of dance when I was in the MFA program at UCLA. I would place a camera in the corner of the studio and whirl and bow for hours, entering trance. Later, I would watch the footage and select movements from the videos that I then shaped into solos and ensemble dances. I still choreograph and source my dances from trance in this way.

What matters most to me is not what I can do, how I can impress, or how great I can appear, but how open I can be to what seeks to move through me. I'm drawn to this because it brings me into communion with the unknown, which is what I dance for. Yet I remain equally rooted in the known: technique, structure, and form. The more disciplined your body, the more you can surrender to the unknowable and serve as its instrument. To enter the heart of chaos and whirlwind and emerge whole requires technique. We are called to become sturdy chalices, able to hold the intoxicating wine of divine grace.

How deeply do you long to be danced, to be guided by something greater? What will you offer in return? How much can you release and step aside, so the greater may move you—and move through you?

100 PERCENT PRESENT AND 100 PERCENT SURRENDERED

It is important to be 100 percent present and grounded and 100 percent surrendered—both fully present and fully gone!

As you let go in the whirling, it may feel chaotic at first, but if you keep turning, order begins to emerge, and you are *danced*. The invitation to us all is: Can you allow that? Can you allow yourself to go to that place of abandon in whatever shape it takes for you, to be birthed into the greater oneness as you?

In trance, you risk your identity, as each experience dissolves more of your illusion of separation from the greater consciousness. And it's not something you direct and create. It *happens* to you. It's grace. Trance is a wild embrace of chaos, a surrender into the arms of the unknown. And that is when—if you are fortunate—you realize, in every cell of your body, the final lesson: the gateway to true embodiment is total surrender, an opening to the love that is already here.

Before I perform, I always pray to be a vessel of the unknowable. On one occasion, I asked in my prayer, "Beloved, I know with my mind that you are everything, but I long to *feel* this truth. I want to taste it and experience in my body. I don't want to hear anything but you!" I went on stage and, to my astonishment, didn't hear a single note the musicians played. It was alarming, but there was nothing to do but surrender. After the performance, the musicians told me they had never seen me dance in such harmony with them. Yet I had not heard a single note they played!

FORTY-DAY SAMA WHIRLING CEREMONY

In 2006, nine years after my first experience in a Sufi Tarighat, I traveled to Turkey to participate in a historic forty-day Sama whirling ceremony, organized by a group of Sufis and guided by the late musician and teacher Oruc Guvenc—peace be upon him—who had decided to follow in the footsteps of Rumi, who is said to have whirled for extended periods, sometimes lasting up to forty days and nights.

There was continuous, glorious music for forty days and nights held in a community of people who shared similar beliefs. I touched many moments of pure bliss during the ceremony—experiences that deepened my dance and spiritual practice. Among the most memorable was the realization that I serve Beauty. My role in the world is to extend the presence of beauty through dance, and to inspire and guide people to feel and embody own beauty as they revere and protect the beauty of the Earth.

Another revelation I had was the experience of Sama as a lovemaking—its sacred ecstatic ripples nourishing not only the whirler herself but the world around her. On one occasion, after hours of whirling, I sat down and, with my eyes closed, reveled in the vast emptiness—the absolute silence of mind that could only emerge after hours of whirling. In that stillness, I heard a woman's voice. Opening my eyes, I saw a veiled woman about my age, seated beside an older veiled woman. The younger one translated for the elder and spoke to me:

"This is my teacher. She leads the Naqshbandi Women Sufis in Istanbul. We were told that there is a woman here making love to Allah, and we came to find her. We see that you are this woman, and we are very happy to have found you."

"Wait, does it really show?!" I asked myself.

I remember that for months after my first forty-day Sama, I was unable to utter any negative words. For the first few weeks, I neither thought nor spoke negatively. Gradually, negative thoughts began to creep back into my mind, but I still could not voice them. They simply would not pass from my lips. After a few months, I found myself again thinking and speaking negatively, but now I could, more or less, observe myself doing so, and it was less automatic. It is said that when you devote yourself to the Beloved for forty days, a spring of wisdom emerges from your heart and flows through your tongue.

Focusing on something for forty days can transform you at a cellular level, with effects far more lasting than a thirty-day concentration. Is there a habit you long to transform by adopting a new practice? Commit to it for forty days, and see what unfolds.

TEACHING AS A WOMAN IN A MOSTLY MALE TRADITION

In 2009, I was honored with the opportunity to teach a workshop in the same Sufi dargah (center—literally meaning "doorway, threshold") where the extended Sama ceremonies were held.

This was a true breakthrough: the first time ever that dance was taught in a traditional Sufi dargah, led by a woman in a largely male-dominated space. Many Sufis draw a distinction between dance and Sama: to them, dance is a presentation, an outward display, whereas Sama is a prayer and a form of meditation.

Rumi, himself, did not make such a distinction. In his poetry, he uses "raghs" (dance) and "Sama" interchangeably. The particular Sufis who were connected with the extended Sama ceremony in Turkey saw my dance as a form of Sama. My heart was lifted as my work of many years was increasingly witnessed and validated as the sacred art I had always dreamed it to be. I had begun to evolve Sama, carrying this ancient and luminous practice into the future.

THE REVOLUTIONARY DIVINE FEMININE SAMA

I resonate with the peacefulness of the traditional Sama, but I mostly whirl in a passionate, volcanic way—a blazing fire rising out of the yin, feminine energy. This is not a negation of how the Mevlevi Sama, with its rules and criteria established by Sultan Valad, has unfolded over the centuries, but rather a progression of it—or perhaps a return to the original way it was danced by Rumi and Shams. "Dancing is not rising to your feet painlessly," says Rumi, "it's about tearing your heart out and scattering it to the four directions . . . the people of God dance in their own blood."[3]

I see my expression of Sama as belonging to the original, wild lineage of Shams and Rumi, as described in Ahmad Aflaki's *The Feats of the Knowers of God*, which recounts the story of Rumi and his disciples.[4] Sama was, and still is, an experiment in the laboratory of integrating spirit and matter. How can it not be unpredictable, wild, at times utterly shattering? The invitation is to give yourself completely to the Beloved so that your body and soul can become one. This is not something you can plan or direct; you can only show up with all that you have so you can be danced.

To dance the Sama, you must be continually engaged in purifying your heart through remembrance—attuning your whole being to the One. My invitation is to marry the transcendent peace of the traditional style with a celebratory ecstasy, offering an initiation into living a sacred and passionate life on Earth.

The Mevlevis turn counterclockwise, but I believe in whirling in both directions. Most of us instinctively prefer to turn toward one direction, and the difference between the two is profound. My understanding of this distinction arises from my own experience up to this moment, not from any claim to objective truth.

Whirling counterclockwise takes you inward, to your deepest core—the point where your identity dissolves into the greater whole. This turn also carries you upward, an evolutionary ascent where body, heart, mind, and soul unite with spirit. Clockwise whirling, in contrast, spirals downward and outward, anchoring you in the Earth so you may embody the revelations of the ascent and offer them as gifts to the world. It is revolutionary—becoming the messenger of the unseen in the seen. One way to understand it is that turning to the left is an initiation into the transcendent Divine Masculine, while turning to the right initiates us into the embodied Divine Feminine.

In our solar system, we have discovered that Venus is the only planet that that rotates clockwise. These explorations take us deeper and deeper, the initiations becoming ever richer as the currents of transcendence and embodiment flow into one another and merge. It is essential to approach the whole endeavor from the realm of mystery. As Rumi says, "Don't look at me with the eyes of the head, see me with the eyes of mystery."[5] The Greek word for mystery, "muo," means "to look with soft eyes." In Sama, we look with soft eyes. Our dance arises from mystery, surrenders to mystery, and vanishes into mystery.

PRACTICE

SURRENDER YOUR HEAD
with video component

This practice opens the gateway of your Throat Chakra, offering a taste of surrender. You may want to have a yoga mat or soft surface to lie on at the end of this practice.

Time required: 5–10 minutes

> Stand or sit on a chair with an upright yet relaxed posture for about two minutes, sensing the ground lovingly through the soles of your feet as you focus your awareness in your throat and neck area. Take a Love Breath.

Ask yourself the following questions, and welcome what emerges:

What lives in this part of my body?

Can I soften enough to be here with ease?

As I listen more deeply, what is my throat longing to share?

After your inquiry, place your hands on your thighs and begin
to swing your head gently from side to side, like a soft whipping
motion. Let the movement radiate like a ray of sun from your
Womb-Dantian, rising through your heart center and into
your neck and head. Once you feel stable and safe: rooted in the
Earth and connected to your Womb-Dantian as the source of the
movement, surrender your head to this side-to-side flow. Allow
it to become light, like a feather. Keep your shoulders relaxed
and still, and feel yourself rooted like a tree from the waist down.
Continue moving your head side to side for as long as it feels good.

Coordinate your movement with chanting "All Love." Chant "all" as
you swing your head to the right and "love" as you swing to the left.

Let your neck move with the rest of your spine. Remember
that your spinal cord begins at your brain stem, so you need to
always keep your neck naturally aligned with the rest of your
spine, to protect both the spinal cord and the cervical vertebrae.

When you are ready to bring the practice to a close, gently
circle your head once in each direction, then come into stillness
and silence. Close your eyes and simply feel your body for a
few seconds without doing anything. seconds without doing
anything. Direct your energy down to your feet.

You may continue sitting or standing, or if possible, lie down
on a yoga mat or a soft carpet. Keep your eyes closed and let

your mind grow quiet. Remain here for as long as you like, welcoming whatever feelings arise without resistance. If you are moved to, let your body stretch in any way that feels nourishing. When you are ready, take a Love Breath, and as you exhale, softly open your eyes.

When you are ready, take a Love Breath and open your eyes as you exhale.

Do not let the weight of your head fall back onto your delicate cervical vertebrae, as this can injure not only the vertebrae themselves but also the discs between them and even the spinal cord. This is why it is essential to initiate the movement from your Womb-Dantian, letting it rise through your heart center before reaching your neck. For a healthy rotation, engage the intercostal muscles of your chest, the muscles of your upper back—including the trapezius—and the supporting muscles of your neck.

∞

PRACTICE

LET YOURSELF BE DANCED
with audio component

This practice invites you to let yourself go and surrender to the music you love.

Time required: at least 5 minutes

Select a piece of music that stirs your heart. Close your eyes and feel the living Earth through your soles. Set the intention to be danced.

With your eyes closed or open, allow the music to move you. Simply dance, letting no thought or distraction pull you away. Do not try to direct the movement—let the movement arise through you.

When the music comes to an end, let your dance come naturally to stillness. Remain in the silence for as long as you can, and simply feel.

If it feels right, pick up your journal and let your experience find its own words—tenderly and without force.

∞

As we release control and let ourselves be danced, a new dimension of awareness opens. The space within and around us comes alive. To whirl is to let go—to dissolve the illusion of control and surrender to being moved by something greater.

The Throat Chakra is the bridge between heart and mind, the place where the voice of the soul can emerge when we release our need to know. Yet this letting go is not confined to whirling alone. It is present in the way we listen deeply instead of rushing to speak, in the way we soften into the rhythm of life rather than resist its flow.

To let ourselves be danced is to trust the unfolding of each moment as if carried by an unseen current, remembering that true joy is born not from control, but from surrender—being danced by the mystery itself. This also translates into daily life, where we learn to loosen the hold of the habitual and open ourselves as a conduit for a greater intelligence to flow within us and through us.

15

EXPAND YOUR VISION

Unearthing the Jewel

*Ray 9: Cultivate Spatial Awareness and Let Dance
Be the Invisible Architecture of Your Vision*

Chakra: 6—Ajna (Authority, Command, or Perceive)

Location: Center of the brain, pineal gland

Anatomical areas of influence: The eyes, pineal gland, brain,
and neurological system

Element: Light

Color: Cobalt blue

Surrender is not only about letting go; it is also about expanding our
awareness. When we release the tight grip of habitual knowing, we
begin to perceive beyond the mind, sensing the space within and
around us as an integral part of the dance. This opening leads us into
the next step of our journey—Chakra 6, the Third Eye, which aligns
with the ninth ray.

One of the most important techniques in Dance of Oneness
related to this ray is learning to be both fully embodied within

yourself and, at the same time, able to observe yourself from above—aware of the spatial patterns you are creating with your movements. Choreography means "drawing in the air." Dance is invisible architecture, and it shows us that our movements not only shape us but also influence the world around us. We are beckoned to create harmonious patterns and spatial designs as we dance, knowing they ripple into our immediate environment and, as our mastery deepens, into the greater world.

Dance also teaches us to become skillful navigators of space, no matter the situation we find ourselves in. To dance your life is to move through every space you enter with an expansive vision and ease, without contracting.

Vision is one of the central capacities of the mind, and to expand your mind is to expand your vision. This is why studying wisdom teachings—ancient and contemporary—that uplift and inspire you, and then embodying them, lies at the heart of Dance of Oneness training. Beautiful, sublime sites in nature can also open your mind, awaken awe and wonder, and raise your frequency.

Our vision is inseparable from what we believe. Believe, and your belief creates reality. All things become possible when you believe. With imagination, you can build images of what you long for—and when you create the image, you give it life. If you can hold it with your mind, you can hold it with your hands and dance it with your body.

It is important to ask yourself what motivates you in making the choices you make. What vision guides your life? Why do you dance, for example? Every choice is a thread in the tapestry of your vision. Consciously or not, you are always creating. The more aware you become of your motivations, the more your actions align with the life you long to live.

UNEARTHING THE JEWEL

I have returned again and again to the question of why I dance, and each time I reconnect with my original vision. A few years before I started the dance MFA program at UCLA, I responded to the resistance I faced from the outside world for pursuing dance by announcing, "I will unearth the dance form I envision from under a great mountain if I have to!" These cryptic words became my actual experience. During the first year of the program, I suffered greatly. I felt like I had to painstakingly excavate every dance I choreographed. I sometimes wish I had said, "I will pursue the dance I'm envisioning as tranquilly and calmly as drinking a glass of water!"

Interestingly, I later learned that "gohar" in Persian means "jewel" or "fire in the Earth"—a hidden treasure waiting to be discovered, while honar (art) is the sacred act of unearthing that jewel, that fire.

OVERCOMING DEEP RESISTANCE

My body was heavy with resistance, and hours of weeping became my inevitable entryway. Voices in my head urged me to stop the disgrace I was bringing upon myself and my family with my so-called "selfish" whims: "What? Do you want to be a whore? Why don't you just stay home or take up a legitimate profession, like becoming a doctor? Why can't you just dance in your living room like so many other girls and women do?"

Other people's voices echoed in me as well, but the ones emerging from inside my own head were infinitely harsher. With every step, I was moving against what had been deeply ingrained in me—an old, cellular imprint carried by women for generations, especially women from the Middle East. "A good woman ought to be silent, submissive, obedient." The shame and the feeling of smallness, of being ridiculed and ostracized, paralyzed me. All I could do was weep and yearn for liberation from the bondage. I knew I had to overcome my paralysis—not just for myself, but for the women of the Middle East and for anyone who has ever felt stunted and unable to express themselves because they had lost touch with their soul.

Despite the techniques I'd learned, the knowledge I'd acquired, and the deep mystical states I'd experienced, I found myself collapsed on the studio floor, unable to move, asking, "Where do you hold back?" The answer was everywhere. I was in chains—bound by habitual thinking, by shame, and by the weight of the world's suffering and injustice. I would go into the studio to create, but within minutes devastation would surface and I would begin to wail. Images and sounds of the world's condition—the cruel, unloving ways we treat one another, ourselves, animals, the Earth, and life itself—together with the traumas of my past, both endured and caused, would flood me, crush and shatter me before I could even take my first steps. How could I possibly express all of that? All I could do was sob and beg for mercy—for a way forward.

I was annihilated by the pain of the world and by the way I held back—the way I would have rather died than open up and express myself. I found the only way I could go forward was to feel the agony fully and let it pierce my heart completely. This initiation, forged in darkness, was a death that led to rebirth. I was in the laboratory of my life, and the experiment was "Express yourself or die!" I died. And from my remains, a tiny sprout broke through—growing into something vast, radiant, and full of promise.

A VISION FOR MY DANCE

I needed to see, to take responsibility, to release, to empty, and to re-pattern through grace. In life, there is sorrow, pain, tragedy, and horror—and these never end. In one of my most desperate moments, lying flat on my back and gripped by psychological paralysis, I suddenly had a vision of myself on a mountaintop soaring high above the Earth. At the center of a vast circular clearing of grass, I was surrounded by Great Souls—Mother Mary, Zarathustra, Rumi, Shams, Yeshua, Miryam the Migdalah, Rabia, Socrates, and countless others. A deep reverence and awe kept me bowed, unable to lift my head and truly see all the beings who were present. Breaking the immense silence, I pleaded, "Please help me. What am I supposed to do?"

"Dance," I heard immediately, "dance to liberate."

The vision gradually dissolved, and I was back in the studio, sprawled on the floor. "Dance! I'm going to dance!" I cried out loud. "I'm going to dance all of it—the joy, the pain, the horror, the deliverance."

Following that voice helped me discover my language. You don't come into the dance already knowing your true language; you must journey toward it—through your life, your soul, your heart, your shattered self and through the dance and movement modalities that meet your deepest spiritual, psychological, and physical needs. All that I perform and teach flowered not only from the techniques and wisdom teachings I had learned and uncovered, but from a resurrection out of utter despair in our shared human condition. This was the final, great recognition on my journey—the one that wove together all the teachings and techniques. It came at the end, born of shattering and a descent into the underworld.

INANNA, QUEEN OF HEAVEN AND EARTH

Life is a dance between the teachings of light and the teachings of darkness. We see this in the myth of the Sumerian Goddess Inanna, who becomes Queen of Heaven and Queen of Earth by plunging into the depths of the underworld—confronting her own shadow, claiming the wisdom of that realm, and extending her love there. She could not be the Queen of Heaven and Earth without her profound understanding of the underworld.

The journey of first becoming fully human and then luminous —which is ultimately the path to becoming sovereign within ourselves—requires venturing into the darkness as a spark of light that gradually grows into a radiant beam. Each of us began in the dark, watery womb of our mothers as a spark of life, unfolding into a fetus. This life we are born into is yet another dark passage, calling us to remember our original spark and, through our own volition and grace, to let it to blaze forth and become a ray of light.

DANCE TO MANIFEST YOUR VISION
with audio component

This practice helps you move from vision to manifestation by embodying your intention through movement. Rather than only imagining
or reflecting on your desire, you will feel it in your body, give it form
through dance, and breathe it into life with your energy. You can do
this practice after the Basic Meditation (chapter 4) or on its own. Have
a yoga mat handy or designate a soft surface to lie on at the end.

Time required: 5–10 minutes

> Select a piece of music you deeply resonate with. Become still,
> connect with your breath, and turn your attention inward to
> your inner eye—the pineal gland (Figure 8), the luminous
> jewel within your brain. Return to this center periodically
> throughout the practice. Long regarded as a gateway between

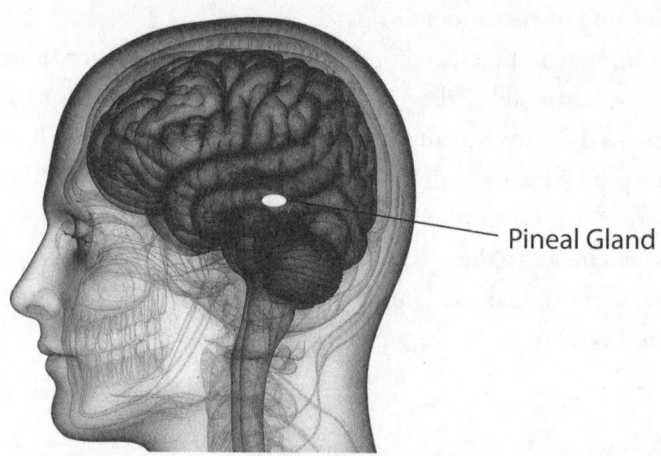

Pineal Gland

FIGURE 8. Visualize your inner eye, the pineal gland in your brain

the metaphysical and physical realms, the pineal gland, when activated, can open you to inspiration and vision while guiding your body and energy field into alignment with that vision.

Ask yourself:

> What is my deepest desire? What do I long to create or become?

See your response with your inner eye. Feel your response in your body as a lived sensation.

Play your music. Speak your vision out loud. Dedicate your dance to it—not as a performance, but as a sacred act of becoming.

Give yourself completely to the dance. Whether slow or ecstatic, let your body give voice to your vision. Through rhythm, gesture, and repetition, you shape energy, moving from passive wishing into active co-creation. Become aware of the patterns and the invisible architecture you are weaving. Explore drawing harmonious shapes in space and notice how they make you feel.

As you dance, feel your vision as real in this moment. This aligns your frequency with its manifestation. Let joy, gratitude, and embodied knowing flow through your movement. Remember, the body does not distinguish imagination from reality—it responds to energy.

After dancing, sit or lie down and let the energy settle. Listen in the stillness.

Ask yourself:

> What small steps can I take now to root this vision in my daily life?

Like planting a seed, dreaming through dance requires ongoing care and return. Each time you dance your vision, you nurture it, refine it, align with it, and breathe life into it.

After the practice, remember to return your attention to your pineal gland throughout the day. Where attention goes, energy flows. The more you attune to this center and grow sensitive to it, the more it activates—opening you to heightened intuition and vision.

∞

Spend time in nature, gazing at awe-inspiring beauty while keeping your focus on your pineal gland. Such beauty nourishes the Third Eye Chakra and expands your vision. As vision expands, you not only become more aware of the space around you—you also begin to see how your beliefs shape your movement and your very existence. What you imagine, you can create. Through belief, you give form to the invisible, allowing inner visions to take shape in the world.

By holding your vision in your mind, you can bring it to life through your body, moving through the world with greater harmony, presence, and grace. As you learn to shape your vision and move through space with intention, you enter into deeper connection with life itself. This awareness invites reverence, a profound respect for the beauty and mystery that surround us.

16

REVERENCE

Flowering into the Unknown

Ray 10: Let Reverence for Life Infuse Your Movement

Chakra: 7—Sahasrara (Thousand-Petaled Lotus)

Location: Top of the head, crown

Anatomical areas of influence: The brain, central nervous system, skeletal and muscular systems

Element: Thought

Color: Violet

When we move with reverence, we acknowledge the sacred and invite it to flow through our body, infusing each step with presence grace. In this chapter, we'll explore the tenth ray of Dance of Oneness and discover how honoring life with reverence opens us to the unknown, allowing us to move with grace, humility, and a profound connection to the great dance of existence itself.

The tenth ray corresponds to Chakra 7, our gateway to spirit and and the greater field of awareness. Here we awaken to the truth that we are individual expressions of the greater consciousness, eternal and connected to all—azali (Persian for "no beginning") and abadi (no end). In this center, we embody the knowing that there is no death, only life—and life is eternal.

Chakra 7 teaches us to live in the present moment. It is only in the present moment that we can access the eternal—where the horizontal axis of time intersects the vertical axis of spiritual ascent, the ney, the rainbow bridge of the chakras.

BEING ALIVE IS A MIRACULOUS MYSTERY

To live fully in the present moment, we are called to release our past experiences. When we keep the past more alive than the present, we obstruct the flow of life force. The present becomes distorted, colored by the lens of what has already happened. Over time, the weight of carrying the past weakens us and can even lead to disease. And yet, we cling to it, mistaking familiarity for security—because the past is known. The present moment, by contrast, is the vast unknown.

Living in the present moment calls for courage, trust, and softening—a willingness to release attachments to habitual beliefs and perspectives. To be truly present, we must let go of old patterns and allow ourselves to be in mystery, open to the new ideas that want to emerge. When our bodies cling to tension or anxiety about the past or future, we block the flow of wisdom available in the present.

Being alive is truly a miracle—pure magic. To receive the fullness of this miracle, we need to be present. Yet many of us become entangled in the past, caught in unresolved emotional or familial wounds, societal pressures, or mental struggles. These experiences can shape our worldview, making it difficult for us to see life as a miracle or our body as sacred. Fear, shame, or a sense of unworthiness can block the awareness of the present moment and all its gifts. We may cling to stories of lack, struggle, or trauma that limit our ability to embrace the fullness of life.

To begin dissolving these blocks, you need to first acknowledge them without judgment. Practice self-compassion, creating space for the present moment. Cultivate gratitude for even the smallest blessings, which can shift your focus from what is missing to what is abundant. Through the practices in this chapter and throughout this book, you can reconnect with your body and reclaim its vitality as part of the miracle of life. Remember: healing and transformation are ongoing processes, and every step—no matter how small—is progress.

If you reflect deeply, you'll find that, the mystery of the unknown is at the heart of everything we think we know. Take our bodies, for example. Like all matter, they are composed of stardust—they are fractal stars. The very atoms and elements that constitute our bodies were forged billions of years ago in the hearts of stars. The carbon, nitrogen, iron in our blood, calcium in our bones, the phosphorous in our DNA—can all be traced to exploding stars, to supernovas. As writer and artist Ella Francis Sanders reminds us, "That particular atom residing somewhere above your left eyebrow? It could well have been a smooth riverbed pebble before deciding to call you home."[1]

REVERENCE

There exists something indisputably greater than us. The openness of the Crown Chakra rests on the fundamental knowing that there is a greater energy moving through us, as us, and through all that is—an energy we didn't create and cannot destroy. It simply is, and we cannot stop it from being.

The seventh chakra is about faith in this greater reality and in all that such faith represents in our lives: inner guidance, devotion and trust. Devotion to something greater is meant to expand us, helping us feel our own greatness—not to contract us into feeling small, nor to elevate us into superiority over those whose faith takes a different form. The energy of the Crown Chakra calls us to seek an intimate connection with the greater presence in everything we do—whatever name we give it: the Divine, Spirit, the quantum field, Love, or the Beloved. Our dance becomes a way of entering this intimate communion. Like authentic prayer and meditation, it is not about turning to the greater for what we can receive, but about turning toward it to be with, and within, a loving presence—to be nurtured and nourished, and reminded of what truly lives in us and longs to live through us. Prayer is less about speaking words to the greater than about living with and as the greater consciousness itself.

Reverence activates the Crown Chakra and plays a central role in Dance of Oneness. When you respectfully acknowledge the sublime beauty of something greater than yourself—that you yourself are a part of and open in awe before its grandeur, you do yourself a profound favor. You generate authentic humility and sincere gratitude, nourishment for the body and soul. By tending to it with devotion, as you would any love relationship, you are nourished in return through the very act of giving attention and care.

PRACTICE

COMMUNE WITH THE UNKNOWN
with audio component

This is a simple inquiry into your relationship with the greater consciousness.

Sit with an upright yet relaxed posture. Close your eyes and feel the living ground beneath you through the soles of your feet. Take a Love Breath, and settle into stillness.

Ask yourself:

Do I believe there is something greater than myself that I am a part of? If so, what is my relationship with this energy—be it Consciousness, the Universe, God, the One, Beloved, Source, or by whatever name I call the Mystery?

How does my relationship with the Greater weave itself into my daily life?

Welcome whatever arises with openness, and allow the
following practice—You Are an Expression of the Greater
Consciousness—to carry these questions deeper into your heart
and psyche.

∞

YOU ARE AN EXPRESSION OF THE GREATER CONSCIOUSNESS
with audio component

Through this practice, you will come to know yourself as an individual
expression of the greater consciousness.

Time required: 45–60 minutes

Begin with the Basic Meditation (chapter 4)

Connect with what animates you—the life force you did not
create but allow to move through you—by tuning into an
awareness greater than your thoughts, emotions, or anything
arising in this moment. You access this by becoming fully
present in your body—by embodying yourself—while remaining
unattached, recognizing that awareness is vaster than the
body. You tune into this greater consciousness as an individual
expression that has taken on form and story. Remember: you are
that greater awareness living this story. Observe yourself from
this spacious, witnessing place with clarity.

When you are ready, bring the practice to a close. Return to this
witness mode throughout your day, observing your habitual
emotions and thoughts from an impersonal stance. The moment

you awaken to the story you have been living, you gain the power to direct it. Life does not have to keep "happening" to you as it has before. If you slip back into believing you cannot direct your story, life will once again resume "happening" to you. Ultimately, it is up to you how much of your story you wish to continue living in the same way.

∞

WALK YOUR DANCE . . . DANCE YOUR WALK
with video component

This practice embodies the ten rays we've explored so far—each one connecting you with the miraculous mystery of life. Before you can dance, you must first learn to walk gracefully, or at least mindfully! The invitation is to dance your walk. In flamenco, for example, the walk itself is everything. A great dancer can move an audience to tears simply by walking across the stage.

As a dancer, you are called to bring your whole being to every moment. When you choose to dance your life, there is no moment in which you are not dancing. It's not that you dance for an hour in class and then rush around the rest of the day like a chicken with its head cut off, tossed about by chaos!

This practice gives you a series of pointers on how to walk with awareness. You can practice at home or in a clearing outdoors, and then begin weaving these techniques into your daily life. If space is limited, walk in a circle. Practice first barefoot, then repeat in shoes.

Time required: 5 minutes

Begin by walking as you normally do, placing your heel down first and rolling through your feet—heel, ball, then toes. Take a few steps this way. Now, see if you can soften your feet, as though you are walking into the Earth rather than on top of her. Let your weight release downward, offering it to the Earth.

Sense the back of your legs, the roots grounding you. Sense your buttocks and your waist. With your awareness, trace up your spine—your tree of life. Sense your lower back, mid-back, and upper back. Sense the back of your shoulders, the back of your neck, and the back of your head. Sense your whole back come alive as you walk, softening your feet into the Earth.

Sense your abdomen. Let your heart lift toward the sky. Imagine an invisible string drawing your head upward as well. It is up to you if you think you end at your head. Continue growing into the sky as you simultaneously soften into the Earth.

Focus on what you are walking upon. Are you walking on the living Earth or on a "dead" surface of some kind? If you are walking on the living Earth, then what do you bring to the Earth in your walk? What do you offer back? Or do you only take, consume, and extract—as humans have done for thousands of years—the story of children who forgot their Mother? Buddhist teacher Thich Nhat Hanh reminds us, "The miracle is not to walk on water. The miracle is to walk on the green Earth in the present moment, to appreciate the peace and beauty that are available now."[2]

When Aphrodite walked, flowers blossomed beneath her feet. As Buddha took his first steps, lotus flowers bloomed under his feet. Imagine flowers blossom under your own. Allow this generative, fertile sensation to flow through your entire body, infusing your gait with ease, sensuality, and grace. Remember to let flowers bloom beneath your feet, especially as you move through man-made, mundane, or stressful places like office buildings, banks, supermarkets, busy streets, or airports. Let your very presence become an act of beauty. Infuse your surroundings with creativity, and walk in service to the Earth, as if each step were a blessing offered to the ground beneath you.

Kiss the Earth as you walk. Feel yourself stepping in peace, in her yin energy, and let the peace enter your body through the soles of your feet.

Become aware of your pace. Soften into the Earth as you ascend into the sky. Focus not only on where you are going, but also on where you are—holding awareness of both. Too often we are so intent on the destination that we bypass the present moment, and life rushes past us at top speed. When you notice yourself hurrying through a stressful situation, slow your pace and attune to the peaceful yin undercurrent of life flowing beneath your feet. In doing so, you will naturally feel greater ease and capacity, and radiate more peace and possibility into the world.

Sense your whole back as you walk and remember to do the same as you stand. We tend to live so frontally, which makes us reactive. Instead, fill the volume of your back and walk with the awareness of your whole back.

Your back is the yang side of your body. Feel it protecting and supporting the front, the yin side. Sense the presence of the Beloved—the support of the universe—always behind you.

As you walk, soften your feet into the Earth, awakening your soles to the living ground beneath you. Sense your vertical alignment extending toward the sky. Sense yourself moving through space with a witnessing awareness, as though watching from outside your body, and feel your connection to the vast, ever-expanding world you belong to. To walk this way is to walk in harmony. The Navajo (Diné) speak of it as walking with the Universe—walking in harmony with all that is. Walk in beauty, attuned to the balance between yourself, the world around you, and the whole of existence. Come in touch with how you are a channel, a bridge between the Earth and the sky. Be in unknowing, for only unknowing expands the mind. All that is known is limited.

When you are ready, bring your walking to a stillness. Close your eyes and observe how you feel.

Practice walking in this vertical, peaceful, exuberant way—sensing all the way up to your crown whenever you remember. Do so especially when you feel tired, low in energy, or heavy in spirit, and notice how it elevates your state.

Remember, with each step you take upon the Earth, you are teaching and transmitting a message. Is it life-affirming—rooted in reverence, love, hope, peace, abundance, and joy—or life-denying, bound to fear, anger, suspicion, scarcity, and despair?

Walking in your most effortlessly vertical posture—rooted in the Earth with peace and rising into the sky with exuberance—is not only for your health and well-being; it becomes an inspiration to others, helping them remember their own radiant verticality. Walking in this way is a living expression of the tenth ray: "Letting reverence for life infuse your movement."

∞

As we move through life with reverence, we deepen our connection to the sacredness of each moment, letting our dance mirror the divine flow. When we honor the unknown with humility and presence, we enter a space where every movement and every breath becomes an offering—an embodiment of the profound mystery that holds us.

Through this honoring, we begin to sense a deeper current—one that guides us toward our true path. When we align with this inner truth, it becomes the ground of our movement, lighting the way forward in the dance of life.

17

THE NORTH STAR

Your Guiding Light

Ray 11: Let True Purpose Be Your Guiding Light and Expression

Chakra: 8—Soul Star

Location: Anywhere from just above the head to roughly one-and-a-half to three feet above it

Anatomical areas of influence: The brain, central nervous system, skeletal and muscular systems

Element: Ether

Color: White or Gold

When we align with this purpose, it infuses every aspect of our being, shaping how we move, dance, and live. In this next part of our journey, we'll explore the eleventh ray of Dance of Oneness and how it brings us into harmony with our true self, guiding us to step forward with intention and authenticity.

The eleventh ray corresponds to Chakra 8, the Soul Star Chakra. Through dance, we awaken to and embody our true calling and purpose. The Soul Star Chakra is the seat of our soul's calling—our North Star.

It is our energetic portal to higher awareness, guidance, and soul-level purpose. It is our connection or gateway to the greater universe, the cosmos, and "all there is." It is the seat of our subconscious mind and interplays with our dream space. In many ways, it is similar to the Crown Chakra, but it is more expansive. Chakra 8 is the transpersonal chakra of unity awareness. Unity awareness is consciousness of the greater whole, of which we are all a part of and now able to embody in human form. Accessing such expanded awareness enables us to transcend the limitations of our human perception and remember that we are not alone, but ultimately are all one.

Rumi asks, "How long will you beg from others, when there are things born of you that emperors desire?"[1] What are the things born of you that emperors desire? The key is to be authentic in your inquiry and response—not just say what sounds appropriate or what you think others will approve of. As the German poet Rilke writes, "Just being here matters, because the things of this world, these passing things, seem to need us to put themselves in our care somehow."[2]

YOUR NORTH STAR IS WHAT YOU ARE PASSIONATE ABOUT

I believe each of us is here to serve an ideal—something we are deeply passionate about—whether love, truth, beauty, goodness, justice, wisdom, peace, freedom, courage, hope, or another guiding force. Our purpose is to expand the energy of what we serve, to remain true to it even in the most difficult circumstances, and to let it guide us through the maze of life, especially when no trace of that ideal can be found in the world around us.

It is essential to trust in what we believe in, even when the outer world offers no support. Rather than giving up or losing faith, we are called to tune into our guiding ideal even more deeply, allowing it to be our North Star.

Your Soul Star watches over you and protects you. The halo above prophets and saints can be seen as a symbol of the Soul Star. It may also envelop you like a mandorla—an almond-shaped frame that surrounds

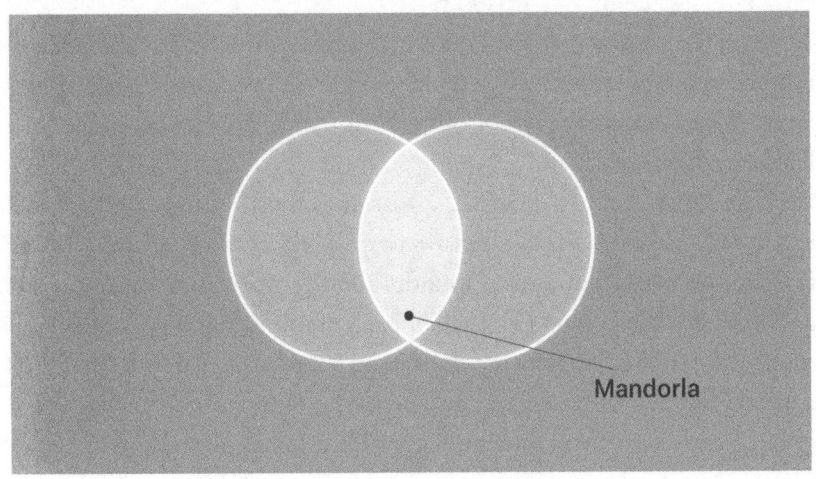

FIGURE 9. The Mandorla is formed by two overlapping circles symbolizing the union of dualities or wholeness

sacred figures. In traditional Christian art, mandorlas often encircle Mother Mary and Yeshua. A mandorla emerges where two circles intersect (see Figure 9). We each have a unique sacred shape or pattern to our Soul Star.

The Soul Star is the seed and origin of the seven chakras in our body. Its energy and influence permeate every center and, by extension, our entire existence. When we attune to it, its radiance can guide and envelop us, illuminating all seven chakras and restoring vitality and hope.

With the Soul Star Chakra, we need to reverse the idiom "seeing is believing" into the deeper truth: "believing is seeing." We have to believe in the Soul Star in order to see it and feel it. We must first believe in something in order to become it.

THE BIRTH OF DANCE OF ONENES

In 1999, as part of my MFA thesis at UCLA, I envisioned a performance that combined live music and dance—a dream seeded in my flamenco days. When I sought collaboration with Iranian musicians, I encountered resistance born of cultural stigma. In Iran, musicians have long been marginalized, while dancers are even lower on the social hierarchy. Many feared that associating with dance would cost them their hard-won legitimacy.

Then I met Pejman Hadadi, a master percussionist who embraced my vision. Together, we created *Amvaaj: Waves from the Unseen*, fusing Persian music and dance in a groundbreaking collaboration. *Amvaaj* was a revelation, challenging entrenched perceptions of dance in Iranian culture. Critics marveled at its depth, though some struggled to reconcile its spiritual essence with its grandeur, believing that true spirituality could only be expressed through simplicity rather than splendor, as the measure of authenticity. Yet for me, sacred dance was exactly that: the union of skill, beauty, and devotion. At last, those around me began to see the vision I had long described. Musicians who had initially refused to collaborate with me exclaimed, "But this is not dance; it is beyond dance!" To which I replied, "No, this is *exactly* dance." *Amvaaj* was more than a performance; it was the embodiment of my purpose, a bridge between dance and spirit.

The success of *Amvaaj* opened doors to international invitations and shifting perceptions in my culture around dance. My relatives, once hesitant about my career, grew proud. Later, collaborating on projects with my father became a joyous cultural celebration of our heritage, and a personal triumph—an honor to be embraced and to create alongside him.

In 2005, I founded Dance of Oneness. My dance had become my prayer, a vessel for embodying the sacred. Teaching this modality was a challenge at first. The professional dance world often resists spirituality, prioritizing form and technique over inner life, while New Age forms tend to elevate feeling over technique and discipline.

Inspired by pioneers like Martha Graham, who called dancers "the messengers of gods,"[3] and Pina Bausch, who sought "what moves people rather than how they move,"[4] I have worked to restore spirit to the art form. In a world where the sacred is misunderstood or undervalued, my mission remains clear: to help people unite spirit and matter through sacred dance, transforming not just movement, but life itself.

My journey is a testament to the power of aligning with true purpose. Even before I began my MFA studies, I met resistance—from my family, from society, and from the cultural stigma surrounding dance. Choosing this path was not easy. Later, when musicians refused to collaborate with me, fearing it would jeopardize their legitimacy, I could have abandoned my vision. Yet something deep inside me knew this was the path I was born to walk. By staying true to my calling, I transformed obstacles into opportunities, creating a new way forward where none had existed—one that has benefited many and influenced dance makers.

I share this because the same is possible for you. When you claim your true purpose as your guiding principle, it becomes a light that illuminates the way—even when the road seems uncertain. Trust it. Let it shine through your dance, your work, and your life. In doing so, you'll not only transform yourself, but also inspire and uplift those around you.

PRACTICE

CONNECT WITH YOUR SOUL STAR
with audio component

This practice helps you connect with your Soul Star. It can follow the Walk Your Dance . . . Dance Your Walk practice (chapter 16).

Time required: 5–10 minutes

> Stand with your eyes closed and sense the living ground beneath your feet. Take a Love Breath. Envision a luminous star above your head, radiating golden or white light. Notice how far above your head it shines, and gently attune to its form—see if you can perceive its shape. Stay with the awareness of your Soul Star for at least one minute.

When you are ready, open your eyes and begin to walk as you did in the Walk Your Dance . . . Dance Your Walk practice. With each step, sense the Earth lovingly beneath your feet. At the same time, feel yourself extending into the sky beyond your Crown, with your Soul Star shining above you. Continue walking with this awareness for two to three minutes.

When you're ready, come to stillness and stand with your eyes closed.

Attuning to your Soul Star, feel a luminous ray streaming from it down into your heart.

Stay in this presence for as long as you wish and meet the following inquiry without overthinking, allowing the responses to emerge from your inner knowing.

Ask yourself:

> What do I love? What do I serve?
>
> What is my purpose in life?
>
> What is my gift or set of gifts connected to my purpose?

Feel the light of your Soul Star bless you and envelop you with its radiance like a mandorla.

When you are ready, take a Love Breath and open your eyes as you exhale.

If you feel moved, take a moment to let your reflections flow into your journal.

∞

Well done! You have ascended through your ney, the reed flute, awakening and activating the eight chakras and the rays of Dance of Oneness that shine through them. You now stand ready for the descent of light—to become a luminous human, a living embodiment of love.

PART III

THE DOWNWARD SPIRAL

Becoming a Luminous Channel of Love

18

BODY OF LIGHT

Living Love

Ray 12: Become Luminous in the Downward Spiral
We have opened in the upward spiral, casting off the veils that obscure our essence, preparing ourselves for the descent of light. We now turn to the final movement of our journey: becoming a luminous channel of love.

To receive the energy of the timeless, we need to attune to our ney and clear it, allowing spirit to flow through us, from infinity above to infinity below. It is no coincidence that Rumi begins his magnum opus, the *Masnavi-ye Ma'navi*, by presenting himself as the ney:

> *Listen to the reed's lament,*
> *as it recounts the tale of separation.*
> *Since the day I was cut from the reed-bed,*
> *my song has moved men and women to weep.*
> *. . . Whoever becomes estranged from their true origin,*
> *longs to reunite with it once again.*[1]

So it is with our own ney, the inner reed. It longs to reunite with its source—the reed-bed from which it feels cut off. The reunion begins when we clear the ney of busy forgetfulness and feel its breath moving endlessly between infinity above and infinity below.

Clarity and freedom may come in flashes of focused practice, yet they call for a lifelong commitment to clearing. The invitation is always to begin where you are. There are countless psycho-physical layers—personal and collective—woven into both body and psyche that you are called to dance through, heal, resolve, and release. You clear what is known so that you may be available to the unknown, and experience yourself as a unique expression of the greater consciousness.

The ney is where you discover liberation from duality. As the central channel of your body, it is not to the right or left, front or back, above or below. So when you hear Rumi's words "I belong to love and am free from both worlds,"[2] think of the ney—where, amidst the noise within and around you, you anchor in stillness and silence.

PRACTICE

RAINBOW MEDITATION
with audio component

This practice guides you to feel the luminous descent—the downward spiral of light infusing your body. You can do this practice after the Basic Meditation (chapter 4) or on its own.

Time required: 5–10 minutes

> Sit or stand in an upright yet relaxed posture. Close your eyes and feel the ground lovingly beneath your feet. Inhale deeply through your nose as you extend your arms out to the sides, then sweep them upward like a snow angel until they meet above your head, palms facing inward. Visualize a white beam of light emanating from the Sun of Love infinitely above, descending toward the crown of your head through the space between your hands.

As you exhale gently through your nose, begin lowering your hands with the palms facing downward. Visualize your Soul Star radiating golden light. The white beam descending from infinitely above transforms into golden light at the level of your Soul Star. Speak your soul's purpose out loud or inwardly. If it is not yet known, listen for it.

Flow with your breath as the light enters Chakra 7, your Crown. Without effort, allow yourself to sense the light changing into violet at the top of your head, establishing your presence in the One.

> Declare: "Beloved, I AM Your extension, here to fulfill my purpose to [fill in the blank]." Feel the radiant crown of your soul's purpose shining upon your head.

As you move your hands down slowly, follow the light as it descends through the ney into Chakra 6—your Third Eye, the pineal gland, your center of vision and inner sight. Watch it turn indigo, and allow this healing radiance to expand into your forehead and eyes, divinizing your vision.

> Say, "I see myself living my purpose," as you visualize yourself living your purpose, surrounded and supported by it.

Flow with your breath and follow the light down into Chakra 5—your throat, your center of will and expression. Watch it turn turquoise, and experience it as liquid, like honey or nectar. Taste its healing sweetness as it fills your mouth, jaw, throat, and neck, divinizing will and expression.

> Say, "In living my purpose, may my words unite rather than divide."

Follow the liquid light into Chakra 4—your heart, your portal to the infinite field of consciousness—and watch it blossom into emerald green. Let this radiance divinize your heart, its healing sweetness flowing through your chest, shoulders, arms, and hands.

> Say, "Beloved, I love You in all people, animals, and life forms. I express my love for You by pouring my love into Your creation. I am grateful for living my purpose." Then feel what it is like to live your purpose, as if it is happening right now. Let joy, appreciation, and gratitude overflow your heart.

Follow the liquid light down your ney into Chakra 3—your upper abdomen, your center of will—and watch it turn yellow. Feel its warmth and sweetness spreading through your abdomen and organs, divinizing your sense of self.

> Say, "I love and honor myself as You, Beloved, and give my all to living my purpose."

Follow the light as it descends into your Womb-Dantian, and notice it deepening from yellow into shades of orange, becoming fully orange in Chakra 2—your genitals and sexual center, the seat of creativity and the balancing of polarities. Let this light fill your hips and genitals with a healing radiance that divinizes your sexuality.

> Say, "I honor my sexuality as sacred, and experience all pleasure as an awakening to You and a delight in You, Beloved. I supercharge my purpose with the exuberant life force."

Follow the liquid light down the ney into Chakra 1—your perineum, your center of connection with the Earth—and watch it turn red. Allow this healing light to saturate the lower part of your hips, buttocks, and legs, streaming through the soles of your feet into the ground, drawing you into a deep resonance with the Earth.

> Say, "I ground my purpose in the Earth and pour this light and my love into the Earth to help regenerate the very place I'm standing upon."

Bring your hands down by your sides. Stand or sit in silence for at least three minutes, feeling the rainbow bridge of light along your ney and radiance filling your whole body. Feel the pulse of your soul's purpose reverberating through you, infusing your being with energy. Hold your focus on offering the light of love into the depths of the Earth, transmitting healing to our glorious planet.

When you're ready to close the meditation, take a few deep breaths, slowly returning to the sensation of your physical body from your feet up to your head. Gently open your eyes when the moment feels right.

∞

You have now awakened the downward spiral of light, connecting deeply with your luminosity. The invitation is to carry this radiance into your everyday life, transforming each moment with presence and purpose. As you anchor this light, you move forward into the pinnacle of our journey, where you will be initiated into uniting matter and spirit through the sacred dance of Sama.

19

SAMA

Grounded Flight

*Ray 13: Unite Matter and Spirit Through
Love and Serve the Greater Good*

You are now ready to be initiated into the sacred dance of Sama, the culmination of all the teachings we have explored throughout this journey. Sama weaves together all the rays of Dance of Oneness. In the heart, the upward spiral of becoming fully human meets the downward spiral of becoming luminous, uniting matter and spirit through love. In Sama, you step into the fullest expression of your divine potential, allowing your being to serve as a vessel for a higher purpose—grounding the light of the Sun of Love in your body and offering it in service to the world.

Everything in the universe spins. The structure of the spin is critical to our understanding of the dynamics of the universe. This is how everything comes to exist. Space-time spins itself into protons, atoms, planets, stars, galaxies, clusters, super clusters, universes, and so on. The spin may be what connects everything together.[1]

Consider all the ways we are spinning: the Earth spins at about 1,000 miles per hour at the equator while orbiting the Sun at 67,000 miles per hour. Our solar system whirls around the Milky Way at 515,000 miles per hour, and our galaxy itself spins through the universe at approximately 1.3 million miles per hour. On the microscopic level, our DNA spirals, atoms spin, and protons turn. How profound then, to enter into the spin consciously—without agenda—simply to be and to listen. Most children delight in spinning; it is an instinctual movement, fundamental to existence itself. Yet as we grow older, many of us fear turning, afraid of losing control. When we learn to trust the spin as a core dynamic of life, we open ourselves to its evolutionary gifts and its power to expand consciousness.

SAMA AND GAMMA BRAIN WAVES

In Sama, we spin ourselves into a unitive state with all that is. We begin to feel the rapture and ecstasy of oneness pulsing in every cell of our body. In the language of neuroscience, this rapture is associated with gamma brain waves. Gamma is a unifying frequency that gives us a profound sense of well-being and connectedness. It supports peak concentration and performance, enhances cognitive functioning, and awakens elevated states of awareness. Experienced meditators often describe it as a "feeling of blessings."

Gamma waves activates unity consciousness—the awareness of the quantum field of energy that connects us to all of life. The ancients knew this field as the Great Mother, who spins, spirals, and weaves the shimmering robe of life in which we live and through which we are connected to all cosmic life.

THE SEVEN INITIATIONS OF SAMA

It is difficult to say when people first began spinning as a dance practice, though it has surely been woven into human life for millennia. In the thirteenth century, Rumi was initiated into Sama by his beloved teacher and spiritual companion, Shams-e Tabrizi. Shams told Rumi that Sama was the only practice he truly needed. Though Rumi had mastered vast knowledge in religion, philosophy, and the sciences, these belonged to the realm of the intellect. Through Sama, Shams assured him, this knowledge would descend into his heart and become integrated into his being.

Sama takes us deeper into the mystery of the birth of the Divine in the human. The very posture of the arms is itself a revelation. In the

Mevlevi Sama, the right arm extends upward with the palm facing up, signifying that one lives by the grace of the light of love. In humble eagerness, the heart receives this light so that, as the left arm extends outward and downward with the palm facing the Earth, the radiance flowing through the heart may be offered to the world. The samazan, or "whirler," turns counterclockwise—toward the left—because this is considered to be the direction of the heart.

The Sufi path to embodiment shines through through Sama, expressed in seven fundamental initiations that lie at the heart of Dance of Oneness.

FIRST INITIATION: Die Before You Die

The first initiation of Sama is the realization that the habitual self you identify as "you" is not your true self, and must be surrendered for you to access your essence—which is none other than the Beloved. The path of living love gives us the strength to allow ourselves to be utterly destroyed by love so we can be recreated in it. This "dying before you die," known in Sufism as fana (annihilation), is echoed in many mystical traditions. We come to see the alchemy of "dying" and "rebirth" into love as the two currents of one miraculous process. Shams says, "Every breath is a chance to be reborn. But to be reborn into a new life, you have to die before dying."[2] Learning how to "die" to the false self is simultaneously learning how to come alive in a fresh, expanded dimension or baqa (life in the Divine). Rumi prays, "Oh Beloved, let this lover die, so it is only you who lives."[3]

Shams taught Rumi that Sama annihilates the false self and liberates us from our two forms of bondage. First, it shatters the illusion of a separate self and all we have come to associate with our self as a fixed entity. Second, it frees us from the false self's fear-based attachment to people and possessions. The more you liberate yourself from these two forms of bondage, the more you align with the Beloved—and with your very essence.

To enter into Sama authentically, is to dance everything other than the Beloved beneath your feet, as the Hindu deity Shiva tramples his demons in the cosmic dance. Your true self blossoms from all that you let die and stand upon—the very forces that once kept you out of alignment with the Divine. When you are no longer ruled by them and can stand firmly upon them, the dramas, deceits, greed, pride, and all impulses not rooted in love become compost, nourishing the flowering of your authentic self.

No practice brings this about as profoundly as Sama. It is the art of opening to hear something greater than the endless chatter of the mind, while also embracing that chatter as part of the journey toward embodying your authentic self. Even beginners often glimpse this transformation. Some of my students, after only a short time whirling, share that they feel a powerful stillness—a taste of the soul. The key is to persevere. The more you whirl, the more this stillness becomes your anchor and center of gravity, around which everything unifies—until its radiance fills your whole being and becomes inseparable from the awareness of who you are.

SECOND INITIATION: Connect Directly with the Source of Inspiration

The second initiation of Sama is the realization that when you empty yourself of "you," you will be filled with the Beloved and connected with the wellspring of creativity. Rumi's love poetry in *Divan-e Shams*—the verses cherished and celebrated across the world—fountained through him in perfect rhyme and meter as he whirled, while his followers faithfully recorded and preserved them. This flowering of poetry is a testament to Sama as an extraordinary meditative dance that aligns us directly with the source of life and the fountain of ever-flowing creativity. Sama unites soul and body, the transcendent and the immanent, the invisible and the visible—bridging them so the Divine may be felt *in* you, *through* you and *as* you.

THIRD INITIATION: Become a Luminous Channel of Love in the World

The third initiation of Sama teaches that when you open yourself to receive the light of the Beloved and allow it to saturate your entire body and being, you naturally begin to radiate that light in your unique expression of love. The more you see and unconditionally honor the radiance of the Beloved in yourself, in other beings, throughout nature, the more you become a channel for divine light in the world. In your presence, all beings instinctively feel their own divinity. The more you mirror the

Beloved in the world, the more vividly you feel the Beloved alive in yourself. It is through transmitting the light of love that you become more radiant and permeated by it.

FOURTH INITIATION: Surrendering to the Unknown

The fourth initiation is this: when you're willing to surrender your habitual grasp on control, a radiant and ever-expanding sense of balance and power can emerge within you—one far beyond what you ever imagined possible. Surrender is not the absence of control; it is yielding to the deeper order already woven into your being. In dancing the Sama, you are brought face to face with your fear of losing control and of falling—a fear most of us resist. Yet this is the only way. The more you are willing to die into life, the more abundantly life can flow through you.

The infinite virtue of Sama is that it dismantles mental chatter. You cannot cling to your identity or memory. You cannot hold onto concepts. You are called to polish your mind and heart like a mirror, and in becoming clear, you begin to reflect the radiance of the unknowable, which shines through you—like the poetry that blazed through Rumi as he whirled.

Can you allow yourself to enter that place of holy abandon, whatever form it takes for you, so that you may be birthed into the greater oneness as the unique expression of yourself? Are you willing to give your all to become the polished mirror through which the light of love streams into the world?

FIFTH INITIATION: Being Simultaneously Empty and Full

The fifth initiation reveals to us that our true identity is found in Laa Makaan (nowhere). In Sama, you experience the no-thingness from which all things arise. As in Taoist philosophy, we come to realize that being flowers from non-being. The Persian phrase "Yeki bood, yeki nabood"—Once upon a time, there was one, and there was no one— beautifully captures this mystery, as do the discoveries of modern physics, which show that the material world emerges from the vacuum, taking form for a moment before returning to it.

In Sama, you die to the separate self (fana) and are reborn in the Beloved (baqa)—simultaneously empty of the self and filled with the Beloved. If your cup is full of yourself, there is no room for the Beloved. But when you are both empty and full, you can dance with the alchemy of opposites: from the ashes of destruction, creation arises; from the depth of affliction, grace emerges.

This is the great paradox: to become everything, you must first be no-thing. You become no one, no body, no thing, no place, no time—so that you may become everyone, every body, every thing, every place, all time: living love.

SIXTH INITIATION: Balance Spirit and Matter

The sixth initiation teaches that embodiment is about balancing spirit and matter in ourselves. Too much light and emphasis on transcendence, and the human aspect drowns and you lose your way in the world. Too much matter, and you become heavy, frozen, overtaken by worries, fears, and "what ifs." Many of us are stuck here.

But wouldn't you rather be open and comfortable in your own skin, exactly the way you are? Only by accepting yourself as you are can you develop the capacity to transform what feels misaligned without being ruled by fear. Sama begins with embracing yourself. First you learn to embrace, and only then can you fly. By trusting, by knowing yourself to be worthy and capable, and by giving yourself fully to the journey, you become ready to take flight.

Through Sama, you enter the true marriage of opposites: between the absolute glory and the absolute mundane, healing the illusion that the miraculous is found only in transcendence and not in the ordinary. In this union, daily life itself becomes luminous. Glimpses of enlightenment may expand you for a time, but when they fade, the ordinary can feel small and contracted. The invitation is to bridge the two worlds—to let the power and glory of spirit permeate matter, infusing every cell of your being, leaving nothing untouched.

SEVENTH INITIATION: Disciplined Ecstasy

The seventh initiation teaches that freedom requires discipline, and ecstasy must be grounded. Alertness, clarity, and rootedness form the essential container for flights into ecstasy—for there is no true flight without grounding. Sama prepares us to be luminous channels of love in the world, and this is a profoundly grounded task.

Rumi inspires us to become a chalice for the wine of divine grace. Sama is intoxicating like wine, yet to prolong its bliss and distill its essence for daily living, you need to be grounded and to cultivate your chalice through disciplined practice. The more you commit to a body-based discipline, the more fully you can surrender to the unknowable and become its instrument. To enter the heart of chaos and whirlwind and survive requires technique—you must become a sturdy chalice able to hold the wine of grace.

Rumi deepens this truth, saying, "The highest state is not drunkenness, the highest state is drunkenness laced with diamantine sobriety."[4] He also says, "May you possess a heart at once drunk yet lucid."[5]

It is important to be 100 percent present and grounded and 100 percent surrendered. Sama is the ultimate experience of being both no-thing and everything, of fusing sobriety with ecstasy. Once you glimpse through grace what can truly take place in Sama and what whirling can initiate you into, you long not only for surrender but also for discipline, so you can experience yourself as living love, surrendered to your transcendent origin.

PRACTICE

INITIATION INTO SAMA
with video component

Prepare an unobstructed space of at least five by five feet so you can turn freely without worrying about bumping into anything. Be sure to practice on an empty stomach, and wear socks or soft-soled shoes so you can slide with ease.

Please note: Everything between "grounding" and "prostrating" is done while spinning. Once you are familiar with the sequence, you may follow the bold instructions as shorthand guidance.

You can whirl with or without music (Please refer to endnotes for a suggested music list[6]).

If you have a disability or are unable to whirl, you can still move through the stages of Sama while in seated meditation.

Time required: Begin with at least 10 minutes, gradually increasing up to 1 hour as you are able.

> **Cross your arms.** Stand with your feet hip-width apart and soften your knees. Place your left arm on your right shoulder and cross your right arm over it, resting your right hand on your left shoulder. This posture carries many meanings; I will share two.
>
> > With this posture, you embrace yourself, vowing to hold whatever arises in this movement meditation in tenderness. The journey toward union with the Beloved begins and ends in an embrace—loving yourself as the Beloved's beloved. First we learn to embrace; only then we can fly.
> >
> > This position also represents the alef (the first letter of the Persian and Arabic alphabets), the primal stroke that signifies the Divine. It is also the number one, symbol of unity. Our aim is to bring body, heart, mind, and soul into oneness, in the name of love. As Rumi says, "Take away one thousand loves and give me the one love."[7]
>
> **Begin with an invocation.** "In reverence to the Divine Presence that permeates all and everything. In recognition of this Presence within myself, in everyone I meet and remember, and in the living Earth. In remembrance and gratitude for the ancestors—all who have carried the light of love into the world on the path of Sama. May Sama illumine my heart and root me deeply in my purpose in the world."

Bow in reverence. Bow your head toward your knees, offering your full reverence to that which you truly revere.

Stay down for a few seconds and savor.

When you are ready, slowly roll up through your spine, one vertebra at a time, with soft knees, your arms in the posture of embrace.

Ground yourself. Stand with your eyes closed, feeling the living Earth beneath your feet. Let your breath flow naturally through your nose, and direct your energy gently down from your head into the rest of your body. Stay attuned to the natural flow of your breath throughout the Sama.

Start to take simple steps. When you're ready, take a step forward with your right foot, keeping your left foot in place.

Next, lift your left heel, pivot on the ball of your left foot, and step with your right foot in a quarter-turn to the left (counterclockwise).

Lift your left heel once more and pivot on the ball of your left foot, stepping into another quarter-turn toward the back, still turning counterclockwise. Repeat this movement two more times to complete a full circle. This is known as a "paddle turn," where your right foot propels the motion and your left foot anchors as the pivot.

Continue stepping in this way. In the tradition of the Mevlevis, this counterclockwise orbit is known as "turning toward the heart." Keep the ball of your left foot rooted to the ground, lifting only your heel as you step with your right foot. This will allow you to remain centered in place.

As the samazan (whirler) learns to whirl, they place the first and second toes of the left foot around a nail hammered into the floor beneath them. This trains them to keep the left foot in place. Imagine this nail in the ground between your two toes, preventing you from lifting your entire left foot off the ground. How fortunate we are in the modern world—we need only to envision the nail rather than risk injuring our toes! The nail is a very powerful imaginary tool for grounding. Dizziness often arises when energy rushes too quickly into your head, and visualizing the nail helps anchor the spin. Many of us are so flighty—accustomed to living in our heads, letting energy rise too quickly upward, or escaping into the transcendent—that we quite literally need to be "nailed" to the Earth in order to be present in the moment! You can also experience the nail as the needle of a compass, held steady by your left foot while your right foot draws a circle around it. In this way, each step inscribes presence into the Earth, while each turn lifts you into the mystery of the heavens.

Try a variation in stepping. Once you feel at ease with the quarter-turns, experiment with half-turns. Begin facing forward.

> Pivot on the ball of your left foot as you paddle with your right foot, making a half-turn to the back.

> Repeat the movement to return to facing forward.

> Continue step-paddling if it feels natural. If not, stay with the quarter-turns and let yourself gradually build toward half-turns.

Look at everything and nothing. Begin by looking directly ahead, then soften your gaze by closing your eyes halfway. This allows you to take in everything and nothing at once, while also turning your gaze inward toward your heart.

Chant to focus. In Sama, the name of the Divine is the point of focus. By chanting the name in your heart or out loud as you whirl, you polish your heart, preparing it to become the home of the Beloved.

> I invite you to chant the name that opens your heart to the Divine—a name like "Beloved." If no name arises, listen inwardly as you whirl. You will know the name is true for you when it steadies and centers you, sustaining you as you spin.

In the words attributed to Yeshua, one can hear an echo of Sama:

> *Oh Birther! Father-Mother of the Cosmos . . .*[8]
> *Focus your light within us—make it useful:*
> *as the rays of a beacon show the way.*
> *Your name, your sound can move us*
> *if we tune our hearts as instruments for its tone.*[9]

Sama is the tuning of the heart to the tone of the One, like an instrument. In this attunement, the name takes root within you, infusing your whole being, moving you, and dancing you. In this way, the voice of guidance resounds through you—just as divine poetry once blossomed from Rumi.

Begin moving your arms. As you turn, slowly move your hands from your shoulders and cross them at the wrists over your heart. Continue turning for several cycles, hands resting there, tuning into the rhythm of your heart.

Bless and release what no longer serves. Identify what you need to release in this moment—what can be cleared and washed from your heart to make space for the Beloved. When you have recognized it, gently uncross your hands and let them descend slowly in front of you, as if clearing and polishing your heart, allowing what you release to flow down into the Earth.

> With your feet, bless and compost what you have released, "trampling," as Rumi says, "everything other than the Beloved under your feet."[10]

> He also says, "Cleanse your chest sevenfold of hate and grudges so that, unto the wine of love, you may become . . .halice."[11]

Grow from your compost. When you are ready, slowly raise your arms in front of you, palms open to the sky, as if following the blossoming of a rose along your ney, tuning into each chakra on the way upward.

Raise your right hand up as a chalice to receive the light. When your arms reach above your head, extend them fully and feel yourself blossoming like a rose into new life. Then open your right palm upward and outward, diagonally into the sky, as you continue stepping and sensing the ground with your feet. This gesture embodies the First Salaam (Greeting): an awakening to the divine origin of all that is, and a declaration that you have been created by Divine power. Raising the right hand toward the sky is your response to the call of love streaming toward us from every aspect of existence, in every moment.

Every moment, from every direction comes the call to love . . .
The dawn of joy is here, the moment of union, of vision.[12]

Shape your right hand as a chalice receiving the light. Let the light flow down your arm and into your heart. As the radiance in your heart grows, you are illumined with a certainty—beyond any possible formulation in words—that all of creation is one with the Creator, and that everything is bound together by the force of love.

Extend your left arm out to transmit the light. Slowly lower it to the side of your body at shoulder level, palm facing down, as you whirl. Shape your left hand like a chalice. Feel the light from your heart flowing through your arm, into your palm, and out into the world—infusing the Earth, all people, and all creatures with the radiance of the Beloved through the love in your heart. Offering to the world the blessings you are receiving from the Beloved in every moment is the essence of the Second Salaam. For it is only in transmitting and giving that you begin to understand and perceive the vastness of the love you are ceaselessly receiving in each and every instant.

The Second Salaam offers one of the most vital guidelines for living. It teaches that loving other beings—people, animals, the Earth herself, and all life forms—is inseparable from loving the Divine and life itself. Each time we look upon another with hatred or animosity, we declare our hatred of the Divine and, in turn, of ourselves—for the way we perceive another is the way we perceive both ourselves and the Divine. This truth holds the key to our healing in these times of intense polarization.

Continue whirling as you chant. Remember, you don't need to *do* anything but simply show up and offer yourself as an open channel.

> If you are stepping in quarter-turns, don't worry about landing precisely in each direction. Keep your attention on your feet, sensing the Earth and the "nail," and let your turn unfold naturally.
>
> If you are stepping in half-turns, stay aware of the forward-and-back rhythm of your steps, yet let your turn unfold naturally. Sense the ground with your feet and feel that with each step you are grounding love in your body and into the world.

Continue whirling for as long as you can. If you are whirling to music, harmonize with its rhythm and let it carry you.

End in prostration. To stop, gradually slow yourself into stillness. Cross your wrists over your heart center, or rest your right hand atop your left upon your heart. Crossing your wrists or arms seals your energy field that has expanded through whirling.

> Once you have come to stillness, bow your head in reverence, as you did in the beginning, and affirm: "All is One."
>
> From there, bend your knees and slowly kneel in prostration, as in the yogic child's pose. Place your palms on the ground beside your head. Touch your forehead to the ground, kiss the Earth, and once more touch your forehead to the ground—offering your reverence to the sacred ground upon which you have been whirling. This posture is called sajdeh (prostration).

Remain in sajdeh for a few breaths, or for as long as feels right for you.

> When you are ready, gently lift your head up from the ground and come to sit—either with your knees together or cross-legged—for at least a few minutes, soaking in the golden silence that follows this glorious sacred dance.

You may then continue with the Basic Meditation (chapter 4) or the Rainbow Meditation (chapter 18).

Sama is a devotional practice through which everything is sanctified and imbued with adoration, rooted in the knowing that the energy of the Beloved is alive everywhere and in everything. Even the smallest acts—like putting on or removing an article of clothing—are done with reverence, each piece kissed as it touches or leaves the body.

Sama is also an ecstatic, trance-inducing, and expansive practice. Give yourself time before transitioning into daily activities—especially driving. To put it simply, you are intoxicated! Yet unlike ordinary intoxication, this leaves no hangover—only a lingering radiance.

Additional Notes and Steps for the Basic Sama

Surrender. Whirling brings you face-to-face with your fears in their helpless nakedness. It reveals that relying on personal strength and the illusion of control—rooted in separateness—is itself the source of fear. At a certain point, you realize the only way forward is complete surrender. Any attempt to direct or control the experience only creates more instability, more dizziness, and thus more fear.

Instead, allow the immensity to penetrate your whole body. The more you surrender, the more ecstatic you become. You may even feel moved to let go fully, pick up the tempo, and joyously cry out the name of the Beloved. The key is to allow yourself to be *danced*.

Understanding the Third Salaam: dying into union. The Third Salaam represents complete annihilation in the Beloved. As you deepen in Sama, you surrender more and more, letting the illusion of a separate self dissolve in the passionate remembrance of the Beloved. Even the most impassioned lover is still conscious of "the self that loves." However illumined by passion, the self still remains. The path of love gives you the strength to allow the separate self to be utterly destroyed (fana) by love, so that you may be recreated within it (baqa). This is the mystery of dying before you die.

To die to the false self is to be reborn in a fresh, expanded dimension of baqa—abiding in the Divine—in the world. "Oh Beloved, let this lover die, so that only You remain," says Rumi.[13]

The garments worn by the samazan (whirler) symbolizes the teaching of the Third Salaam. The hat represents a tombstone, while the white dress recalls the Persian tradition of wrapping the corpse in a white shroud before placing it in the grave.

Experiment with the full Mevlevi turn. Once you have danced the Sama on several occasions, you may wish to explore the full turn—the way a Mevlevi samazan turns. After becoming comfortable with half-turns, begin stepping into complete turns by pushing off with your right foot while pivoting on the ball of your left foot. Step forward with your right foot each time. Let these complete turns arise naturally from the half-turns, rather than forcing them.

You may also experiment with tilting your head to the right. The Mevlevi samazan turns with a tilted head so the eyes follow the heart. The tilt also symbolizes fana. Interestingly, the Earth itself rotates on a tilt in its counterclockwise orbit—much like a Mevlevi samazan!

Understanding the Fourth Salaam: love in action. The first three Salaams are journeys to the Beloved that culminate in fana—the dissolution of the separate self. The Fourth Salaam is the never-ending journey *in* the Beloved, or baqa. The true whirler does not retreat from the world; they serve it. They become a lighthouse in the storm, a ray of the sun shining into darkness—not with judgment, but with love. The aim of the Sama is not only to taste trance-like bliss, but to live a human-Divine life as the Beloved in action—serving the evolution of all beings and the Earth through love. Rumi says, "How long do I want to revel in ecstasy? Let me bring others to ecstasy."[14]

The more you dedicate yourself to whirling on a regular basis and the more you surrender all of your knowing to the mystery, the more the treasures you uncover in Sama will shape your daily life. You begin to embody the resonance of "I AM love in action." Listen deeply as you ask the Beloved to guide you in serving at your highest potential, in reverence to the Earth. Sufi mystic Sheikh Ansari describes the Fourth Salaam beautifully:

> *Beloved, grant me eyes that behold only Your Radiance.*
> *Gift me a mind that delights in serving You.*
> *Fill my heart with the wellspring of gratitude to pour forth.*
> *Bless me with life that I may dedicate it to the healing of*
> *   the world . . .*[15]

As we whirl, we enter a state beyond thought. The habitual mind grows quiet. Time stretches—or disappears. We become pure sensation, pure presence. The separate self dissolves, and in that dissolution, something greater emerges: the soul, the light-body, the part of us that has never been apart from the Source. We do not become light in some abstract metaphorical way; we literally grow more luminous. Our cells vibrate at a higher frequency, our nervous system recalibrates into harmony, and those around us feel it. In this state, we do not just receive love—we transmit it. We become a mirror of the Sun of Love: steady, unconditionally generous, and unwavering.

Experiment with whirling clockwise. Everyone instinctively favors one direction over the other. While the whirling darvishes traditionally turn counterclockwise—toward the heart—every direction can open us into heart-centered presence. I invite you to try turning clockwise and notice how it resonates with you. The key adjustment is to visualize a nail rooted in the ground between the first two toes of your right foot, using your left foot to step—or "paddle." Your arm positions can remain the same. For a deeper understanding of the symbolism of clockwise and counterclockwise whirling, refer to chapter 14.

∞

Now you have learned how to ground your soul in your body, to experience the infinite within the finite, and to become a luminous channel of grace and love in action in the world, as an individual expression of the greater consciousness. You have entered into the ancient cosmic dance that connects you directly with the creative source of the universe—your divine origin—and opens space for the Beloved to live in you and express through your unique way of living love, in reverence to the Earth.

Now, you have come full circle, and I invite you to "let your dance unfold"[16] and open yourself to embodying the deathless consciousness of the divine human: love.

CONCLUSION

Finding Joy in Divine
Play and Service

As we bring this journey together to a close, I want to leave you with the essence of what we have explored: the invitation to live your life as a dance—to experience the sacredness of your own body as a channel for the greater consciousness, and to open to the joy of being a living expression of love.

Dance is a way to embrace joy, integrate pain, and return to the simple, innate pleasure of being alive. It reminds us that life itself is divine play, and our bodies are the vessels through which this dance unfolds. At the heart of Dance of Oneness is the joy of lila, a Sanskrit term for "divine play." Across many spiritual traditions, creation is seen as a cosmic dance, a radiant unfolding in which we are not merely spectators, but active participants. Yet this dance is not for our personal joy alone. As we deepen into presence and awaken to who we truly are, a natural yearning arises to serve, uplift, and share the light we have kindled with all beings.

THE DANCE OF BEING

We often think of joy as a fleeting emotion, something that comes and goes depending on external circumstances. But the kind of joy I'm speaking of here is something deeper. It is a state of being that arises when we allow ourselves to be fully present in our bodies and fully engaged with each moment as an expression of love. It is the joy of being an instrument of the Beloved, in harmony with the rhythms of life.

We have explored how dance can bring us into this alignment. Whether by moving energy through the spirals in the ney or awakening light within the body, these practices are not ends in themselves; they are sacred tools for remembering our wholeness and reconnecting with the web of life. Through this wholeness, we discover joy, not as a personal possession, but as a state of communion. And from this communion comes the call to serve the greater good.

PLAY AS MEDICINE

Many of us have been conditioned to view life as a series of tasks, responsibilities, and struggles. In this paradigm, play is often seen as frivolous or childish—something that must be left behind as we grow older. But what if play was not an escape from reality, but the medicine we need to heal from heal from life's heaviness? What if play was the very essence of the Divine?

Through dance, we reclaim play as a sacred act. Dance reminds us that life is not meant to be conquered, but to be experienced, savored, and celebrated. In this way, play becomes joyful medicine.

And from this wellspring of joy arises the natural desire to wish happiness for all beings—to lift others as we rise. Joy becomes complete only when it is shared. True joy is the joy of giving, of seeing another smile, of knowing that your actions contribute to the collective awakening and healing of the world.

DANCE AS A PATH TO LIBERATION AND COLLECTIVE AWAKENING

In the same way that dance can be medicine, it can also be a path to liberation. The word "liberation" often evokes images of freedom from something—freedom from suffering, from limitations, from oppression, etc. But liberation is also the freedom to express yourself fully, to live in alignment with truth and to experience the fullness of life without holding back.

Rooted in the Divine Feminine lineage of Dance of Oneness, the practices in this book have prepared you for a sacred task: to birth a new humanity grounded in love, reverence, and interconnection—beginning with yourself. This is a humanity that honors the body as a luminous temple, recognizes the Earth as holy, and embraces all beings as kin. The Divine Feminine reminds us that liberation is not an escape from the world, but an embodied presence within it. Through these practices, you have cultivated your capacity to midwife this new humanity. Each time you move with intention, breathe with awareness, or hold space with love, you are actively bringing this birth closer.

THE JOY OF UNION

One of the most profound gifts of dance is the experience of union. In dance, we come into union with ourselves, with each other, with the Earth, and with the Divine. We touch the truth that we are not separate beings moving through a fragmented world, but interconnected expressions of the same life force. This union is not something to be attained; it is our natural state. Through dance, we simply remember.

And from this union flows the most natural expression of the awakened heart: service. Service to others. Service to beauty. Service to love. Service to joy. When we live in this way, our joy becomes a blessing—a ripple that extends outward, uplifting all of life.

THE INVITATION TO CONTINUE THE DANCE

Beloved dancer, I invite you to carry the essence of this journey into your daily life. Dance and practice regularly. Let your body be a vessel for joy, for healing, for divine play, and for loving service. Remember that dance is always available to you, especially when life feels uncertain or heavy. When you approach life as a dance, you cultivate the resilience to meet challenges with presence and grace.

Remember to play, remember to serve. Remember to wish happiness and freedom for all beings. Know that each time you choose love, each time you choose to dance your life, you uplift not only your spirit, but also the greater web of existence, helping to birth a new humanity— one that remembers and loves.

Step into the flow, and let the joy of divine play carry you forward, ever closer to the truth of who you are, as you awaken love and joy in others.

The dance is eternal. And you are an essential part of it.

ACKNOWLEDGMENTS

I bow in gratitude to my father, Parviz Sayyad, and my mother, Parvin Mahdabi, for gifting me life and instilling in me the courage to live it fully, and to my sister Maryam, whose presence has been a constant source of love. I honor my grandmother, Batool Abedian Salimi, my first spiritual teacher, who has passed into the realm of spirit yet remains ever-present in my heart, and the eternal spirit of Rumi, whose teachings continue to illuminate my path. I am deeply grateful to my dear friend Andrew Harvey, who encouraged me to write this book, to my agent Anne Marie Farrell, who believed in it from the beginning, and to the great team at Sounds True for carrying it into the world. Above all, I thank my students, who are the heartbeat of this work and the reason it lives and breathes, and you, dear reader, for opening your heart to walk this path with me. May this book be an offering of love and light in service to the awakening of all beings.

NOTES

INTRODUCTION
1. Jalal al-Din Rumi, *Divan-e Shams*, translated by Coleman Barks in an intimate gathering of friends in Los Angeles on May 22, 2017.
2. Jalal al-Din Rumi, *Masnavi-ye Ma'navi*, translated by Banafsheh Sayyad.
3. Jalal al-Din Rumi, *Masnavi-ye Ma'navi*, translated by Banafsheh Sayyad.

CHAPTER 1
1. Jalal al-Din Rumi, *Divan-e Shams*, translated by Banafsheh Sayyad.

CHAPTER 2
1. Daniel Matt, *The Essential Kabbalah: The Heart of Jewish Mysticism* (San Francisco: HarperOne, 2009), p. 24.
2. Anne Baring and Jules Cashford, *The Myth of the Goddess: Evolution of an Image* (London: Penguin Books, 1993), p. xi.
3. René Descartes, *Discourse on Method and Meditations on First Philosophy*, translated by Donald A. Cress (Indianapolis: Hackett Publishing, 1998), p. 18.
4. Andrew Harvey and Anne Baring, *The Divine Feminine: Exploring the Feminine Face of God Around the World* (Berkeley: Conari Press, 1996), p. 10.
5. Jude Currivan, *The 8th Chakra: What It Is and How It Can Transform Your Life* (Carlsbad, CA: Hay House, 2006), p. 12.
6. Amit Goswami, *The Self-Aware Universe: How Consciousness Creates the Material World* (New York: Putnam, 1993, p. 30).
7. Malcolm Carter, *The Connected Universe* (Vancouver: The Connected Universe Film, Inc., 2016).

8. Lao Tzu, *Tao Te Ching*, translated by Stephen Mitchell (New York: HarperCollins e-book, 1988), chapter 4.

9. Imam Bukhari, *Sahih Bukhari*, translated by Dr. Muhammad Muhsin Khan (Riyadh: Darussalam, 1997), Book 76, Hadith 319.

10. Andrew Harvey and Eryk Hanut, *Perfume of the Desert: Inspirations from Sufi Wisdom* (Wheaton, IL: Quest Books, 1999), p. 73.

11. Some Sufi teachers and mystics might not consider adab the third central practice on the Sufi path. They point instead to other principles, such as futuwwa—spiritual chivalry, the code of honor and generosity.

12. Jalal al-Din Rumi, *The Essential Rumi*, translated by Coleman Barks (San Francisco: HarperOne, 1995), p. 36.

13. Lao Tzu, *Tao Te Ching*, translated by Stephen Mitchell (New York: HarperCollins e-book, 1988), chapter 28.

CHAPTER 3

1. Andrew Harvey and Anne Baring, *The Divine Feminine: Exploring the Feminine Face of God Around the World* (Berkeley: Conari Press, 1996), p. 6.

2. Çatalhöyük is a very large Neolithic and Chalcolithic proto-city settlement in southern Anatolia, near Konya, which existed from approximately 7500 BC to 6400 BC and flourished around 7000 BC, first excavated in modern times around 1958. The discovery of many statues of a Mother Goddess deity in this site suggest that a Goddess-based culture existed here.

3. *Surah Al-Ikhlāṣ* (Sincerity, Devotion), Chapter 112 of the Quran, translated by Banafsheh Sayyad.

4. Jalal al-Din Rumi, *Divan-e Shams*, translated by Banafsheh Sayyad.

5. Anne Baring, "The Shekinah-Sophia: Divine Wisdom and the Holy Spirit," paper presented during the *Madonna Rising Virtual Intensive* (Ubiquity University, 2020), p. 7.

6. Andrew Harvey, *Turn Me to Gold: 108 Poems of Kabir* (Unity Village, MO: Unity Books, 2018), p. 163.

7. Jalal al-Din Rumi, *Divan-e Shams*, translated by Omid Arabian; *The Universe in You* (Los Angeles: YOUniversal Center, 2014), p. 36.

8. Anne Baring, "The Two Marys of Chartres," paper presented during *Madonna Rising Virtual Intensive* (Chartres: Ubiquity University, 2019), p. 3.

9. Jehanne De Quillan, *The Gospel of the Beloved Companion: The Complete Gospel of Mary Magdalene* (Ariège: Éditions Athara, 2010) p. 60.

10. Jalal al-Din Rumi, *Masnavi-ye Ma'navi*, translated by Banafsheh Sayyad.

CHAPTER 4

1. Jalal al-Din Rumi, *Masnavi-ye Ma'navi*, translated by Banafsheh Sayyad.

2. Inscription on the External Temple of Luxor, Egypt, ca. 1400 BCE (Luxor, Egypt).

3. Inscription on the Internal Temple of Luxor, Egypt, ca. 1400 BCE (Luxor, Egypt).

4. Jalal al-Din Rumi, *Masnavi-ye Ma'navi*, translated by Banafsheh Sayyad.

5. Markus MacGill, "Oxytocin: What Is It and What Does It Do?" *Medical News Today*, September 21, 2015, beauty.medicalnewstoday.com.

6. Markus MacGill, "Oxytocin: What Is It and What Does It Do?," *Medical News Today*, September 21, 2015, beauty.medicalnewstoday.com.

CHAPTER 5

1. Jalal al-Din Rumi, *Divan-e Shams*, translated by Banafsheh Sayyad.

2. Nassim Haramein, *Quantum Revolution*, video series on Gaia, 2020, gaia.com.

CHAPTER 7

1. Martha Graham, *Blood Memory* (New York: Doubleday, 1991), p. 115.

2. Tantra is an esoteric yogic stream that arose in the Indian subcontinent beginning in the mid–first century CE, taking root within both Hindu and Buddhist traditions.

3. The Bible, *Luke* 23:34.

4. Jalal al-Din Rumi, *Divan-e Shams*, translated by Banafsheh Sayyad.

5. Daniel C. Matt, *The Essential Kabbalah: The Heart of Jewish Mysticism* (San Francisco: HarperOne, 2009), p. 63.

CHAPTER 8

1. Neil Douglas-Klotz, *Prayers of the Cosmos* (New York: HarperCollins, 1990), p. 60.

2. Mantak Chia, *Awakening Healing Energy Through the Tao: The Taoist Secret of Cultivating Internal Power* (Santa Fe: Aurora Press, 1991), p. 33.

3. Neil Douglas-Klotz, *Prayers of the Cosmos* (New York: HarperCollins, 1990), p. 59. This is the translation from the original Aramaic of Matthew 5:7 in the Bible, which is typically translated as "Blessed are the merciful, for they will be shown mercy."

4. Caroline Myss, *Anatomy of the Spirit: The Seven Stages of Power and Healing* (New York: Random House, 1996) p. 83.

5. Jalal al-Din Rumi, *Divan-e Shams*, translated by Banafsheh Sayyad.

6. Caroline Myss, *Anatomy of the Spirit: The Seven Stages of Power and Healing* (New York: Random House, 1996) p. 169.

7. Jalal al-Din Rumi, *Divan-e Shams*, translated by Banafsheh Sayyad.

8. Gitta Mallasz, *Talking with Angels*, translated by Robert Hinshaw (Einsiedeln: Daimon Verlag, 1988), p. 230–231.

9. Gitta Mallasz, *Talking with Angels*, translated by Robert Hinshaw (Einsiedeln: Daimon Verlag, 1988), p. 231.

CHAPTER 9

1. Clarissa Pinkola Estés, *The Creative Fire* audiobook (Louisville, CO: Sounds True, 1991).

2. Clarissa Pinkola Estés, *The Creative Fire* audiobook (Louisville, CO: Sounds True, 1991).

3. Jalal al-Din Rumi, *Divan-e Shams*, translated by Banafsheh Sayyad.

4. Jalal al-Din Rumi, *Divan-e Shams*, translated by Omid Arabian; *The Universe in You* (Los Angeles: YOUniversal Center, 2014), p. 42.

5. Jalal al-Din Rumi, *Divan-e Shams*, translated by Banafsheh Sayyad.

6. Federico Garcia Lorca, "*Theory and the Play of Duende*," translated by A. S. Kline, poetryintranslation.com, 2007, p. 8, 17.

7. Jalal al-Din Rumi, *Divan-e Shams*, translated by Banafsheh Sayyad.

CHAPTER 10

1. Lao Tzu, *Tao Te Ching*, translated by Stephen Mitchell (New York: HarperCollins e-books, 1988), chapter 8.

2. Jalal al-Din Rumi, *Divan-e Shams*, translated by Banafsheh Sayyad.

3. Lao Tzu, *Tao Te Ching*, translated by Stephen Mitchell (New York: HarperCollins, 1988), chapter 14.

4. Malcolm Carter, *The Connected Universe* (Vancouver: The Connected Universe Film, Inc., 2016).

5. Jalal al-Din Rumi, *Divan-e Shams*, translated by Banafsheh Sayyad.

CHAPTER 11

1. George Ivanovich Gurdjieff, "Sayings of Gurdjieff," *Gurdjieff International Review*, gurdjieff.org.
2. Jalal al-Din Rumi, *Divan-e Shams*, translated by Banafsheh Sayyad.
3. Alejandro Jodorowsky, *The Spiritual Journey of Alejandro Jodorowsky* (Rochester: Park Street Press, 2008), p. 262.

CHAPTER 12

1. Jalal al-Din Rumi, *Divan-e Shams*, translated by Banafsheh Sayyad.
2. Jalal al-Din Rumi, *Divan-e Shams*, translated by Banafsheh Sayyad.
3. Jalal al-Din Rumi, *Masnavi-ye Ma'navi*, translated by Banafsheh Sayyad.
4. This data is based on research by the HeartMath Institute.

CHAPTER 13

1. Jalal al-Din Rumi, *Masnavi-ye Ma'navi*, translated by Banafsheh Sayyad.
2. Jalal al-Din Rumi, *Masnavi-ye Ma'navi*, translated by Banafsheh Sayyad.

CHAPTER 14

1. Jalal al-Din Rumi, *Divan-e Shams*, translated by Banafsheh Sayyad.
2. Jahanshah Ardalan, *Beyond Words*, documentary film, 2003.
3. Jalal al-Din Rumi, *Divan-e Shams*, translated by Banafsheh Sayyad.
4. Shams al-Din Ahmad Aflaki, *Manaqeb al-arefin* (The Feats of the Knowers of God), translated by John O'Kane (Leiden: Brill Academic, 2001).
5. Jalal al-Din Rumi, *Divan-e Shams*, translated by Banafsheh Sayyad.

CHAPTER 16

1. Ella Francis Sanders, *Eating the Sun: Small Musings on a Vast Universe* (New York: Penguin Books, 2019), p. 1.
2. Thich Nhat Hanh, *Touching Peace* (Berkeley: Parallax Press, 2005), p. 11.

CHAPTER 17

1. Jalal al-Din Rumi, *Divan-e Shams*, translated by Banafsheh Sayyad.
2. Rainer Maria Rilke, *Duno Elegies*, translated by Gary Miranda (Portland: Tavern Books, 2013), p. 68.
3. Martha Graham, *Blood Memory* (New York: Doubleday, 1991), p. 5.

4. Pina Bausch, quoted in Norbert Servos, *Pina Bausch: Dance Theatre* (Munich: K. Kieser, 2008), p. 12.

CHAPTER 18

1. Jalal al-Din Rumi, *Masnavi-ye Ma'navi*, translated by Banafsheh Sayyad.
2. Jalal al-Din Rumi, *Divan-e Shams*, translated by Banafsheh Sayyad.

CHAPTER 19

1. Malcolm Carter, *The Connected Universe* (Vancouver: The Connected Universe Film, Inc., 2016).
2. Shams al-Din Tabrizi, *Maghalat-e Shams-e Tabrizi*, translated by Banafsheh Sayyad.
3. Jalal al-Din Rumi, *Divan-e Shams*, translated by Banafsheh Sayyad.
4. Jalal al-Din Rumi, *Divan-e Shams*, translated by Banafsheh Sayyad.
5. Jalal al-Din Rumi, *Divan-e Shams*, translated by Banafsheh Sayyad.
6. Ömer Faruk Tekbilek, album: *Whirling* (Tucson: Celestial Harmonie, 1994); Homayoun Shajarian, Sohrab Pournazeri & Siavash Ensemble, album: *The Lords of the Secrets* (Oakland: Mystic World Music, 2015).
7. Jalal al-Din Rumi, *Divan-e Shams*, translated by Banafsheh Sayyad.
8. Neil Douglas-Klotz, *Prayers of the Cosmos* (New York: HarperCollins, 1990), p. 12.
9. Neil Douglas-Klotz, *Prayers of the Cosmos* (New York: HarperCollins, 1990), p. 16.
10. Jalal al-Din Rumi, *Divan-e Shams*, translated by Banafsheh Sayyad.
11. Jalal al-Din Rumi, *Divan-e Shams*, translated by Banafsheh Sayyad.
12. Jalal al-Din Rumi, *Divan-e Shams*, translated by Banafsheh Sayyad.
13. Jalal al-Din Rumi, *Divan-e Shams*, translated by Banafsheh Sayyad.
14. Jalal al-Din Rumi, *Divan-e Shams*, translated by Banafsheh Sayyad.
15. Sheikh Ansari, *Al-Maqsad al-Asna*, translated by Banafsheh Sayyad.
16. Jalal al-Din Rumi, *Divan-e Shams*, translated by Banafsheh Sayyad.

ABOUT THE AUTHOR

Banfsheh Sayyad is an Iranian spiritual embodiment teacher, sacred dancer, choreographer, and activist. She is the founder of Dance of Oneness®, a Divine Feminine lineage rooted in dance as a spiritual path, and the science of embodiment, uniting three streams of transformation: the art of dance—rigorous technique and self-expression—holistic healing, and wisdom teachings.

Banafsheh is among the few bearers of authentic Persian dance in the world. She has been dancing the Sufi Sama for thirty-five years and is a pioneer in creating a liberated feminine expression in a genre long performed only by men.

With easeful instruction and a welcoming spirit, Banafsheh empowers students from all seasons of life to feel a deep sense of belonging in their bodies and passion in their lives. Her signature style of holy wildness, infused with ancient wisdom, awakens transformation and illumination in all who dance with her or witness her art.

Banafsheh holds an MFA in Dance from UCLA, a master's degree in Chinese medicine, and her award-winning work has been presented across North America, Europe, and Australia. Her acclaimed dance film with Andrew Harvey, *In the Fire of Grace*, traces Rumi's journey of the soul through movement. Banafsheh's website is danceofoneness.org.

ABOUT
SOUNDS TRUE BOOKS

Sounds True was founded in 1985 by Tami Simon with a clear mandate: to disseminate spiritual wisdom. Since starting out as a project with one woman and her tape recorder, Sounds True has grown into a mission-driven learning and media company, partnering with many of the leading wisdom teachers and visionaries of our time.

Every Sounds True Book is designed to not only provide information to a reader but to also to embody the quality of a wisdom transmission, unlocking our greatest capacities to love, serve, and uplift others.

Sounds True Books are part of St. Martin's Essentials, an imprint of Macmillan Publishers.